QUESTIONS
& ANSWERS
FROM
CLINCAL MEDICINE

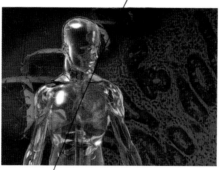

*For Elsevier*

*Commissioning Editor*: Ellen Green/Pauline Graham
*Development Editor*: Clive Hewat
*Project Manager*: Kerrie-Anne Jarvis
*Designer*: George Ajayi
*Illustration Manager*: Merlyn Harvey

# 1000 QUESTIONS & ANSWERS

## FROM
## CLINICAL MEDICINE

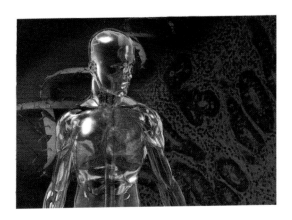

### Professor Parveen Kumar CBE BSc MD FRCP FRCP (Edin)

Professor of Clinical Medical Education, Barts and the London, Queen Mary's School
of Medicine and Dentistry, University of London, and Honorary Consultant
Physician and Gastroenterologist, Barts and The London NHS Trust and the
Homerton Hospital NHS Foundation Trust, London, UK

### Dr Michael Clark MD FRCP

Honorary Senior Lecturer, Barts and the London, Queen Mary's School of
Medicine and Dentistry, University of London, UK
Consultant Physician Princess Grace Hospital, London

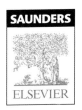

**SAUNDERS**

ELSEVIER

Edinburgh London New York Oxford Philadelphia St Louis Sydney Toronto 2008

# SAUNDERS

## ELSEVIER

© 2008, Elsevier Limited. All rights reserved.

No part of this publication may be reproduced, stored in a retrieval system, or transmitted in any form or by any means, electronic, mechanical, photocopying, recording or otherwise, without the prior permission of the Publishers. Permissions may be sought directly from Elsevier's Health Sciences Rights Department, 1600 John F. Kennedy Boulevard, Suite 1800, Philadelphia, PA 19103-2899, USA: phone: (+1) 215 239 3804; fax: (+1) 215 239 3805; or, e-mail: healthpermissions@elsevier.com. You may also complete your request on-line via the Elsevier homepage (http://www.elsevier.com), by selecting 'Support and contact' and then 'Copyright and Permission'.

First published 2008

ISBN: 978-0-7020-2886-1

**British Library Cataloguing in Publication Data**
A catalogue record for this book is available from the British Library

**Library of Congress Cataloging in Publication Data**
A catalog record for this book is available from the Library of Congress

**Notice**
Knowledge and best practice in this field are constantly changing. As new research and experience broaden our knowledge, changes in practice, treatment and drug therapy may become necessary or appropriate. Readers are advised to check the most current information provided (i) on procedures featured or (ii) by the manufacturer of each product to be administered, to verify the recommended dose or formula, the method and duration of administration, and contraindications. It is the responsibility of the practitioner, relying on their own experience and knowledge of the patient, to make diagnoses, to determine dosages and the best treatment for each individual patient, and to take all appropriate safety precautions. To the fullest extent of the law, neither the Publisher nor the Authors assumes any liability for any injury and/or damage to persons or property arising out or related to any use of the material contained in this book.

*The Publisher*

The Publisher's policy is to use **paper manufactured from sustainable forests**

Printed in China

# Contents

# Acknowledgements

We would like to thank everyone who has helped in the preparation of this book – especially Ellen Green, who originally commissioned the book from the source questions and answers on the *Clinical Medicine* website, and other Elsevier staff – Pauline Graham, Clive Hewat, Kerrie-Anne Jarvis, George Ajayi, and Caroline Cockrell. We are also grateful to Ms Jillian Linton, and Sue Beasley who helped prepare the manuscript, and to the copy-editor Eleanor Flood.

# Preface

This book is the result of some of the questions, which you, the readers of *Clinical Medicine*, have sent to us. We have changed some of the earlier answers to bring them up to date but, in general, we have tried to keep the book as authentic as possible. It is therefore not a complete coverage of all that is in *Clinical Medicine*. A number of your questions were quite penetrating, raising issues that were quite unusual. All were a challenge to answer. We hope you like this small book and find it useful in answering the many intriguing questions that are presented to you by patients every day.

We would like to thank all the authors of *Clinical Medicine* who, with their hard work in producing coherent chapters, made this book possible. We would also like to thank all of you who have sent in questions; these are always extremely helpful in making changes to the new editions of *Clinical Medicine*.

Finally, please continue to feedback your questions and comments to us. We find them extremely valuable.

*PJK*
*MLC*

# Ethics and communication 1

## QUESTIONS

### Question 1
Regarding medical ethics, if a man is discovered to be hepatitis B or C positive, is it advisable for the physician to inform the wife or sexual contact of the patient?

### Question 2
Is it unlawful in most countries to limit medical care, particularly by rationing the usage of drugs? Surely rationing must be against the oath we took as doctors to provide the best care available.

### Question 3
What is meant by QALYs? Is there a difference between quality and quantity of life?

### Question 4
Are 'Do not resuscitate' orders illegal in most countries?

### Question 5
What is a living will?

### Question 6
I've heard of the Bolam principle but when I mentioned it to my lecturer I was told it was out of date. Could you explain please?

### Question 7
Why is counselling required before an HIV test can be done on a patient? We don't counsel patients when we look for a tumour marker to diagnose cancer, which is often more serious for a patient.

## Question 8
As a junior doctor, I have to attend many multidisciplinary team meetings. I am concerned about the confidentiality of these meetings as they are attended by a diverse group of healthcare workers.

## Question 9
Is the role of the advocate in a medical interview to help the patient or the doctor?

## Question 10
We are always asked by our seniors to make sure that the patient has signed the consent form. Isn't verbal consent enough? Also, for what procedures do I have to get consent, e.g. urinary catheterization in a patient with retention?

# ANSWERS

## Answer 1
No. The doctor can only give confidential information to the patient. One would expect, however, that the doctor would counsel the patient, giving advice on his sexual behaviour and safe sex. The patient would hopefully discuss the results with his partner.

## Answer 2
In all healthcare systems, rationing has become inevitable, partly because of the high costs of modern therapies. To be in line with good medical practice, doctors must acknowledge the obligation that, if rationing is unavoidable, it should be carried out in a responsible and justifiable way.

## Answer 3
QALYs are Quality Adjusted Life Years. These were developed to place a measurable value to the quality and quantity of life. They were used to try and assess the value of different health measures. More recently, the value of 'quantity' over quality has been re-emphasized, i.e. a long life of diminished quality could be as worthwhile as a short life of high quality.

## Answer 4
It is accepted in most countries that 'futile' treatment should not be offered. However, all decisions must be made by senior medical staff after discussion with a patient (if competent), other members of the team and family/carers (if the patient lacks mental capacity).

## Answer 5
This is a written advanced directive made by competent persons prior to incapacitation, when they would be unable to express their wishes for treatment, resuscitation and terminal care, e.g. to refuse tube feeding if they were to become unconscious from a stroke.

## Answer 6
Following the Bolam case (*Bolam* v. *Friern Hospital Management Committee* 1957), a doctor is not guilty of negligence if he or she has acted in accordance with a practice that is accepted as proper by a responsible body of medical personnel skilled in that particular art. More recently, it was held that for a judge to rely on the opinion of a medical expert, the judge has to be satisfied that the expert's opinion has a logical basis (*Bolitho* v. *City and Hackney Health Authority* 1997). This means that judges can now reach their own conclusions.

*Further reading*
Kumar P, Clark M (2005) Clinical Medicine, 6th edn. Edinburgh, Elsevier Saunders, pp. 1–18. Schwartz L et al. (2002) *Medical Ethics*. Edinburgh, WB Saunders.

## Answer 7

In the early days of HIV, AIDS was an inevitably fatal condition. It was therefore thought wise to obtain permission and counsel the patient prior to the test. Highly active antiretroviral therapy (HAART) has changed this but counselling is still thought necessary. Your second point is very valid but opinions might change.

## Answer 8

Your patients must always be informed about the meeting. It should be emphasized that modern medicine involves people from many disciplines. It must be made clear to patients that their confidentiality will be preserved within the team.

*Reference*
Fleissig A et al. (2006) Multidiscplinary teams in cancer care. *Lancet Oncology* 7: 935–943.

## Answer 9

Both! However, an advocate represents the values, interests and desires of patients and speaks on their behalf. She or he protects their rights, helps with consent, protects patients' autonomy and ensures that they receive their fair share of resources. From a doctor's point of view, it is nice to have someone who can interpret patients' needs.

## Answer 10

The law in the UK is clear: touching a patient without prior permission is assault or battery. It is therefore essential that the consent (with an explanation of what will be done) is clearly written down and signed. In view of this, really every procedure should have a written consent. However, the Courts will accept the concept of implied consent for minor procedures, such as venepuncture. The example you give is in a grey area and, if in doubt, always get written consent.

*Further reading*
Federation of Royal College of Physicians of the UK (FRCP) (2004) *Good Medical Practice for Physicians*. London, FRCP.
General Medical Council (GMC) (2006) *Good Medical Practice*. London, GMC.

# Infectious diseases, tropical medicine and sexually transmitted infections 2

## QUESTIONS

**Question 1**
Which haematogenous infections (bacterial, fungal and protozoal) can give rise to positive findings in the urine? What are the appropriate microbiological investigations for each infection?

**Question 2**
Could you please explain the term 'zoonosis'.

**Question 3**
What are soil transmitters?

**Question 4**
Please explain the difference between bacteraemia and septicaemia. Can the presence of toxins, fungi or viruses in the blood also be called septicaemia?

**Question 5**
I want to know about the safety of antibiotics used in pregnancy in different trimesters.

**Question 6**
What are the uses and the side-effects of the antibiotic lincomycin?

**Question 7**
I have a question that keeps troubling me. Is there any drug taken orally that prevents penicillin hypersensitivity reactions?

**Question 8**
Is there any replacement intravenous antibiotic for those patients who have hypersensitivity to penicillin?

## Question 9
Is it correct to perform an intradermal skin sensitivity test before administering penicillin or a cephalosporin?

## Question 10
Why are antibiotics not allowed in the treatment of rotaviruses?

## Question 11
Does aciclovir prevent the chances of developing herpes zoster (shingles) when given during primary infection?

## Question 12
How long does it take after vaccination to become immunized against chickenpox and therefore safe to work in infectious areas?

## Question 13
Is meticillin-resistant *Staphylococcus aureus* (MRSA) the only major hospital-acquired infection?

## Question 14
Do you have to have antibiotics to get *Clostridium difficile* infection?

## Question 15
Why do some patients with rheumatic fever later progress to chronic rheumatic heart disease?

## Question 16
What is the World Health Organization recommendation for the prophylaxis of rheumatic fever after a streptococcal throat infection?

## Question 17
Does rheumatic fever have an infectious or an immunological aetiology?

## Question 18
Why is migratory polyarthritis found in rheumatic heart disease?

## Question 19
Are penicillins still the drug of choice in streptococcal infections (particularly *Strep. Pneumoniae*)?

## Question 20
1. How long can the antistreptolysin-O (ASO) titre remain positive after a streptococcal infection?
2. What is the effect of a suitable antibiotic on the ASO titre, if any?

## Question 21
What is the correct method of diagnosis of meningococcal septicaemia: cerebrospinal fluid culture or blood culture?

## Question 22
Can *Escherichia coli* 0157 be spread by foods other than meats?

## Question 23
I have a question about a patient with brucellosis in whom, after 6 weeks of treatment with 600 mg rifampicin +200 mg doxycycline, the agglutination test still shows a 1/320 titre. If, after stopping the treatment, the patient begins to experience identical symptoms as previously, how should treatment proceed? What is the best laboratory test to show relapse?

## Question 24
Do steroids have a role in the treatment of dengue haemorrhagic fever, in particular to prevent the further fall in the platelet count?

## Question 25
Please give me the mechanism of thrombocytopenia in dengue and malaria.

## Question 26
What is the recommended procedure for the treatment of a case of dengue fever?

## Question 27
What diseases can you get from tick bites?

## Question 28
Why has severe acute respiratory syndrome (SARS) not spread as widely as was predicted?

## Question 29
Please explain the relation between recurrent typhoid fever and chronic carrier, and the recommended treatment for both.

## Question 30
What is the single most confirmatory diagnostic test for typhoid?

## Question 31
Has human-to-human transmission of the H5N1 avian influenza virus been described?

## Question 32

In brucellosis, is it possible to see a brucella agglutination test of more than 1/160 even for years after specific and successful therapy of brucellosis?

## Question 33

Please define the terms holoendemic, mesoendemic, and hyperendemic in relation to malaria.

## Question 34

You only recommend malarone for malarial prophylaxis when there is a significant chlorquine resistance. Isn't malarone now widely used in travellers going to areas with low resistance.

## Question 35

Parenteral vaccination with a killed suspension of *Vibrio cholerae* is recommended by some – isn't an oral vaccine better?

## Question 36

Please suggest possible reasons why *Entamoeba histolytica* infection associated with bloody diarrhoea is not relieved by treatment with ciprofloxacin and metronidazole 400 mg × 2 daily over a 3-week period.

## Question 37

Is there a basis for treating patients for filariasis according to the eosinophil count (except for cases of tropical pulmonary eosinophils; TPE)? Filariasis is everywhere in my part of the world; a fluorescent antibody test (FAT) might not be very useful – except when there are very high values.

## Question 38

Why do patients who ingest eggs from a tapeworm in contaminated food not develop tapeworms?

## Question 39

I have a query about one of the details in the book. You mention that perihepatitis is a feature of gonorrhoeal infection, but other books say that perihepatitis (Fitz-Hugh–Curtis syndrome) is a complication of chlamydial infections. Is there a possibility of perihepatitis in gonorrhoea? Thank you.

## Question 40

In the 6th edition of Kumar and Clark *Clinical Medicine*, you indicate that there is no benefit in treating the male partner of a woman diagnosed with bacterial vaginosis (BV). As many physicians use the 2 g × 1 metronidazole dose, is this unwarranted? Does it differ in women experiencing frequent recurrences of infection?

## Question 41
Why is a caesarean section recommended for the delivery of HIV-positive women?

## Question 42
Why is HIV not transmitted when delivering a baby through caesarean section?

## Question 43
1. Is HIV transmitted from mother to child during breastfeeding?
2. Is it possible to be infected with HIV through the ingestion of food and drinks contaminated with the virus?

## Question 44
Is it true that some patients are resistant to HIV infection despite repeated exposure to the virus?

## Question 45
With regard to live vaccination and HIV, can MMR be given to an HIV-positive baby?

## Question 46
In a patient with meningitis: can the development of digital gangrene of the thumbs and sudden dyspnoea with a respiratory rate of 40/min, with intercostal, subcostal and suprasternal withdrawal, be attributed to disseminated intravascular coagulation (DIC)?

## Question 47
1. What are the causes of anaemia in HIV infection?
2. What are the measures necessary to prevent the transfusion of HIV-infected blood to an individual (please explain in light of the window period)?

## Question 48
What is the recommended treatment for pulmonary anthrax?

## ANSWERS

### Answer 1
Haematogenous infections seldom give rise to positive findings in the urine. However, infections such as infective endocarditis do produce red cells in the urine. On the whole, microbiological investigations of the urine are not useful in haematogenous infections.

### Answer 2
Zoonoses are infections that can be transmitted from wild or domestic animals to man. Infections are acquired in various ways, e.g. direct contact (rabies from a dog bite), ingestion of animal products (campylobacter from chickens) and via an arthropod vector (tick bite, Lyme disease).

### Answer 3
These are helminth infections and the main ones are ascariasis, trichuriasis and hookworm.

### Answer 4
'Bacteraemia' means viable bacteria in the blood, e.g. viable bacteria can be found after tooth extraction. The term 'septicaemia' is difficult to define and is being replaced by 'systemic inflammatory response syndrome' (SIRS) (*see K&C 6e, p. 968*). By definition, this implies that at least two of the following are abnormal:
- temperature ($>38°C$ or $<36°C$)
- heart rate ($>90$ beats per min)
- respiratory rate ($>20$/min or $PaCO_2 < 4.3$ kPa)
- white blood cell count ($>12$ or $<4 \times 10^9$/L or $>10\%$ immature forms).

SIRS has many causes; bacterial infection is the most common.

### Answer 5
Antibiotics, like all drugs, should be avoided in pregnancy if possible. Co-trimoxazole is thought to be a teratogenic risk in the first trimester and produces neonatal haemolysis in the third trimester. Quinolones should also not be used in pregnancy. Whenever one is prescribing an antibiotic it is always wise to check local antibiotic policy, and this is even more so in pregnancy. Some drugs are not known to be harmful in pregnancy, e.g. penicillin.

### Answer 6
Lincomycin is not available in the UK; its uses and side-effects are similar to those of clindamycin (*see K&C 6e, p. 39*). Its main use is in osteomyelitis because it is concentrated in bone.

## Answer 7
In the rare situation that no other antibiotic is available, steroid therapy would be the best measure to prevent hypersensitivity reactions. Penicillins, cephalosporins or any other beta-lactam antibiotic should not be used in patients with a history of penicillin allergy.

## Answer 8
Yes, erythromycin is a good IV alternative, e.g. in severe respiratory tract infections. Vancomycin is used IV in serious infections caused by Gram-positive bacteria. There are some other examples but which antibiotic is used depends on the type of bacteria. Note that 10% of penicillin-sensitive patients will also be allergic to cephalosporins.

## Answer 9
No, it is unhelpful.

## Answer 10
Rotavirus is a virus and therefore is not sensitive to antibiotics, which are used for bacterial diseases.

## Answer 11
There is no evidence that giving aciclovir during the primary infection (chicken pox) has any effect on the subsequent development of shingles.

## Answer 12
To ensure safety for healthcare workers in this situation, antibody levels should be checked 1–2 weeks post-vaccination.

## Answer 13
No. Vancomycin-insensitive *Staphylococcus aureus* (VISA), vancomycin-resistant *Staphylococcus aureus* (VRSA) and glycopeptide-resistant enterococci (GRE) are also problems. *Clostridium difficile* is another problem and occurs mainly after taking antibiotics.

## Answer 14
Yes. *Clostridium difficile* is normally carried by approximately 5% of the healthy population. It can cause diarrhoea after other normal bowel commensals have been eliminated by antibiotics. In addition, debilitated patients on antibiotics might be infected by the faecal–oral route. Patients and healthcare workers can spread the organism through hand contact, hence the importance of hand washing.

## Answer 15

Antibodies to streptococcal polysaccharides are substantially elevated and can cross-react with some myocardial tissue antigens. The pathogenesis is, however, far from clear.

## Answer 16

Phenoxymethylpenicillin 250 mg twice daily until the age of 20 years or for 5 years after the latest attack. This prevents recurrence and further cardiac damage.

## Answer 17

Both. Rheumatic fever starts with a streptococcal sore throat. It is followed by an immunological response, which is the result of molecular mimicry between the M proteins of the infecting *Streptococcus pyogenes* and cardiac myosin and laminin. This causes the cardiac lesions. Also, see next answer.

## Answer 18

Migratory polyarthritis found in rheumatic fever is due to the reaction of the circulating M protein of *Streptococcus pyogenes* and the synovial membrane. It is therefore migratory. There is no long-term damage to the joints.

## Answer 19

Penicillin (usually amoxicillin) is the drug of choice for streptococcal infections. However, resistance to *Streptococcus pneumoniae* is increasing (up to 25% in some studies) and you should check your hospital's antibiotic policy for the appropriate antibiotic.

## Answer 20

1. The ASO titre peaks 4–5 weeks after infection. The levels then fall rapidly with a slower decline after 6 months.
2. Antibiotics have no effect on the levels.

## Answer 21

Blood culture for meningococcal septicaemia. For treatment and vaccination see Box 2.1.

---

### Box 2.1 Meningococcal septicaemia

- Minutes count! Give IV penicillin immediately.
- Meningococcal vaccination: travellers to Saudi Arabia for the Hajj and Umrah pilgrimages must receive the polysaccharide vaccine (A, C, W 135 and Y serogroups).

## Answer 22
Yes. The reservoir for *Escherichia coli* 0157 is mainly the intestines of cattle. Thus, pasture land can become contaminated and organisms can be found on vegetables, e.g. sprouts and lettuce; unpasteurized milk is another source.

## Answer 23
Significantly raised agglutination titres can remain for 2 years so these are not useful in diagnosing a relapse. Blood culture (positive in 50%) or polymerase chain reaction (PCR) should be used.

## Answer 24
Two randomized, controlled trials (RCTs) in children have shown no benefit in children with dengue haemorrhagic fever. No effect was observed on bleeding episodes, other complications or mortality. Fluid replacement is vital.

*Further reading*
Wills BD et al. (2005) Comparison of three fluid solutions for resuscitation in Dengue shock syndrome. *New England Journal of Medicine* **353**: 924.

## Answer 25
- Dengue: platelet destruction due to virus/antibody immune complexes binding to the platelet surface. There is also a direct toxic effect on bone marrow.
- Malaria: cytokine suppression of haemopoiesis.

## Answer 26
Mild cases need no active treatment. Dengue haemorrhagic fever requires urgent treatment, the key element being fluid replacement.

*Further reading*
Kumar P, Clark M (2005) *Clinical Medicine*, 6th edn, p. 54. Plus online appendix: http://www.studentconsult.com
Wills BA et al. (2005) Comparison of three fluid solutions for resuscitation in dengue shock syndrome. *New England Journal of Medicine* **353**: 877–889.

## Answer 27
Lyme disease is well known in the West. Other diseases include tick-borne relapsing fever (*Borrelia* spp.), Rocky mountain spotted fever (*Ricketssia ricketsii*), Mediterranean spotted fever (*R. conorii*), Ehrlichosis (*Ehrlichia* spp.) and babesiosis (*Babesia* spp.).

## Answer 28
SARS is due to a previously unknown coronavirus. The reservoir includes civet cats, racoons, ferrets, badgers and animals that are sold in

some Chinese food markets. Strict control of this practice has brought the epidemic under control but it might well return unless regulations are tightly monitored.

*Further reading*
Guan Y et al. (2004) Molecular epidemiology of the novel corona virus that causes severe actue respiratory syndrome. *Lancet* **363**: 99–104.

## Answer 29
A chronic carrier is a patient who continues to carry the organism, usually in the gall bladder, for several months after clinical recovery. A 'carrier' implies no symptoms. A recurrence of disease occurs because of reinfection.

## Answer 30
Blood culture, which is positive in up to 80% of cases.

## Answer 31
Human-to-human transmission is rare at the moment and most cases have been from transmission from birds and animals. The concern is that efficient transmission between humans will become substantial with changes in viral antigenicity.

*Further reading*
World Health Organization (2005) Review. Avian influenza A (H5N1) infection in humans. *New England Journal of Medicine* **353**: 1374.

## Answer 32
Yes. Agglutination levels of 1/160 can persist for years. A four-fold rise in titre is needed to make a diagnosis of acute infection.

## Answer 33
These terms are defined in terms of the parasitaemia rate in adults or palpable spleen rates in children 2–9 years of age:
- hypoendemic is less than 10%
- mesoendemic 11–50%
- hyperendemic 51–75%
- holoendemic greater than 75%.

## Answer 34
Yes, you are correct. The main problem with malarone is its expense. Remember, no drug is 100% effective. Always use insect repellents and insecticide-treated nets at night. Always check on the likelihood of chloroquine resistance in the country you are going to visit.

## Answer 35

Yes. Injectible cholera vaccine provides unreliable protection and is not available in UK. Oral vaccine containing inactivated Inaba strains (including El-Tor) and Ogawa strains is much better. However, this does not mean that precautions with the local drinking water should not be undertaken.

## Answer 36

We can't easily explain this; metronidazole is very effective in invasive amoebiasis. The most likely reason is that in this patient the diagnosis is wrong and you're dealing with another cause of bloody diarrhoea (e.g. inflammatory bowel disease) and the *E. histolytica* is present in the stool of your patient who is a carrier (i.e. not cause and effect).

## Answer 37

The definitive diagnosis is made by demonstrating microfilariae in the blood but absence does not exclude the disease. Eosinophilia is usually present during the acute phase of inflammation, so in the correct clinical context this could be used as a guide to treatment.

## Answer 38

To get tapeworms you need to ingest cystercera (not eggs), usually from eating undercooked pork. If you eat tapeworm eggs, as a result of faecal contamination of food, human cysticercosis might occur.

## Answer 39

Fitz-Hugh–Curtis syndrome was originally described as a complication of gonorrhoea infection, which still occurs. Chlamydia infection is now a much more common cause.

## Answer 40

Placebo-controlled trials have shown that treatment of the male partner does not improve clinical outcome of treatment of BV or reduce recurrences. These trials included the use of metronidazole. The current guidelines do not recommend treatment of male partners. BV does seem to be acquired sexually so the reason for the lack of benefit of treatment is obscure.

## Answer 41

HIV is shed into the cervical/vaginal birth canal as well as being present in the blood, which is why caesarean sections were used. However, with the use of highly active antiretroviral therapy (HAART) during pregnancy, the viral count is low and there is now no advantage in doing a caesarean section.

### Answer 42
HIV is transmitted by blood and not usually by other fluids. There is very little contact between the baby and blood in a caesarean section.

### Answer 43
1. Breast-feeding doubles the risk of mother-to-child transmission of HIV infection.
2. No.

### Answer 44
Yes, it is true but only in a very few patients. One explanation is that mutations in the gene expressing the receptor for chemokine CCR5 (*see K&C 6e, p. 133*) might impair entry of HIV into cells and therefore confer some resistance to infection.

### Answer 45
Yes, but not while the baby is severely immunosuppressed.

### Answer 46
This sounds like meningococcal septicaemia, which can occur with meningococcal meningitis. It could be due to DIC, which certainly occurs, but the best clinical evidence of this is subcutaneous haemorrhages, gastric bleeding or bleeding from venepuncture sites.

### Answer 47
1. One of the most common causes is related to highly active antiretroviral therapy (HAART), e.g. megaloblastic anaemia, red call aplasia with zidovudine. Always remember to check drug therapy and side-effects. Other causes include anaemia of chronic disease and pancytopenia secondary to overwhelming opportunistic infection.
2. In 2000, an assay for HIV RNA was introduced into blood-donor screening. HIV RNA appears earlier than p24 viral protein or HIV antibody. The window period is now thought to be 6–38 days. Transfusion of 'window-period' blood probably accounts for all HIV transmitted by transfusion in developed countries.

### Answer 48
Ciprofloxacin IV 400 mg twice daily. Untreated, the mortality rate is 90% and even in recent cases treated with ciprofloxacin for 60 days (in the USA) the mortality rate was still 45%.

# Cell and molecular biology, and genetic disorders 3

QUESTIONS

### Question 1
As cells grow and regenerate, what mechanism does the body use to get rid of the continuously dying cells? And what kind of cells can't be replaced once dead?

### Question 2
I cannot find out why some of the autosomal dominant diseases have a male or female preponderance, e.g. I have never seen a female Marfans. I was attributing it to imprinting but on reading about imprinting in detail it cannot be the case.

### Question 3
We have been told that some tumours in the colon are associated with microsatellite instability. What does this mean?

### Question 4
I understand that microarrays are being used to define the molecular abnormality and the prognosis in some patients with leukaemia. What are microarrays?

### Question 5
Why do mitochondrial diseases cause a myopathy?

### Question 6
Why do successive generations of patients with some genetic disorders present earlier and with progressively worse symptoms.

## ANSWERS

### Answer 1
Cells are continually dying by a process of apoptosis (programmed cell death). These cells (or their fragments) are phagocytosed by macrophages or neutrophils where they undergo autolysis within these phagosomes. Brain cells cannot be replaced when dead, although recent evidence challenges this view.

*Further reading*
Voss H. V. et al (2006) *Journal of Clinical Investigation* **116**: 2005–2011.

### Answer 2
By definition, the genes responsible for autosomal dominant diseases must be located on the 22 autosomes; thus both males and females are affected. Males and females are affected in equal proportions except in sex-limited disorders, e.g. ovarian cancer with BRCA1 locus.

### Answer 3
Microsatellites are short sequences of randomly repeated segments of DNA, two to five nucleotides in length. These regions are inherently unstable and susceptible to mutations. They have been found in tumours, notably colonic, particularly in individuals with hereditary non-polyposis colorectal cancer (HNPCC).

### Answer 4
Microarrays are, as you say, used to analyse gene expression. The technique is a significant advance because thousands of genes can be screened at any one time. The assays works by using a fluorescently tagged known mRNA, binding to the specific DNA template from which it originated. The amount of bound mRNA can be measured accurately.

### Answer 5
Muscles derive energy via oxidative phosphorylation. Mutations in mitochrondrial DNA impair oxidative phosphorylation.

### Answer 6
This process is called 'genetic anticipation' and is due to expansion of the trinucleotide repeat within the disease gene with each generation. It has been shown in, for example, Huntington's disease (CAG) and dystrophia myotonica (CTG).

# Clinical immunology 4

### Question 1
Please could you explain how lymphocytes (especially B) can maintain receptors on their surfaces? Is this genetically related? If so, when the lymphocytes are first exposed to the antigens, how could the antigen receptor be synthesized?

Is there a mutation within the nuclei of these lymphocytes when they learn to make the receptors? If there is, can you explain how this occurs?

### Question 2
I understand how nuclear factor-$\kappa$B (NF$\kappa$B) works in the inflammatory response but what is the mechanism by which it causes cancer?

### Question 3
What are the diseases associated with hypocomplementaemia and which complement deficiency in particular?

### Question 4
What is meant by 'B lymphocytes are sensitive to clonal deletion'?

### Question 5
What are the immunological implications of 'bare lymphocyte syndrome'/MHC deficiency?

### Question 6
Please explain oligoclonal and monoclonal.

### Question 7
I was wondering if there is any study regarding cell culture techniques of CD4 helper cells (stem cell culturing) and, if so, is it of any benefit to HIV-infected patients?

## Question 8
How do you define autoimmune disease?

## Question 9
1. Why is dexamethasone not routinely used instead of prednisolone, which is almost universally used routinely in autoimmune diseases, or other indications for steroids? Is it because dexamethasone lacks the mineralocorticoid activity seen with prednisolone and therefore does not cause salt/water retention and hypertension?
2. Can high doses of dexamethasone be used in acute relapses of multiple sclerosis (MS) in place of pulse methylprednisolone? If so, what is the recommended dosage?

## Question 10
What is meant by 'pus cell' and is this term synonymous with neutrophils?

## Question 11
Can dendritic cells migrate into lymph nodes? Immunology textbooks state that these initial blood monocytes infiltrate inflamed tissue. Is the professional antigen-presenting cell the dendritic cell that enters lymph nodes?

## Question 12
1. How often should treatment with azathioprine be monitored with liver enzymes and a full blood count?
2. What is the most specific liver enzyme or function test for monitoring azathioprine therapy?

## Question 13
Do you agree or disagree that the dose of azathioprine should be adjusted according to the dose that lowers lymphocytes to $0.8 \times 10^9/L$?

## ANSWERS

### Answer 1
B cells differentiate from lymphoid cells in the bone marrow in a way that allows them to express an antigen receptor on the surface permanently. The expression of the receptor is a definition of B cells and is a result of the differentiation pathway. The antigen receptor varies from one immature B cell to another. There are billions of different receptors, but any B cell will express only one type of receptor. The antigen does not 'design' the receptor; rather, a clonal B cell that recognizes the antigen (very few B cells will recognize a given antigen) will proliferate in response to the antigen and signals from T cells.

As the B cells proliferate and differentiate further, the DNA region that codes for the antigen receptor undergoes mutation, and cells with mutations that recognize the antigen better are selected for further development, while those that do not recognize the antigen die.

### Answer 2
NFκB is a transcription factor that alters cell behaviour. It inhibits apoptosis and increases cell proliferation by increasing the production of tumour necrosis factor (TNF-$\alpha$).

### Answer 3
The following are the major patterns of deficiency:
- C3, C1q and factors H and I: susceptibility to capsulated bacteria, also systemic lupus erythematosus (SLE)-like syndrome
- C5-9: susceptibility to disseminated neisserial infections
- C1 esterase deficiency: hereditary angio-oedema.

(*See K&C 6e, p. 217* for a discussion of complement deficiency.)

### Answer 4
Clonal deletion occurs during the development of immune tolerance (*see K&C 6e, p. 216–217* for a detailed explanation). Clonal deletion occurs when lymphocytes of a particular specificity are lost when in contact with 'self' or an extrinsic antigen.

### Answer 5
In the bare lymphocyte syndrome, a rare recessive condition, major histocompatibility complexes are not expressed. The clinical manifestation is of severe combined immune deficiency (SCID). Patients present in infancy with viral, bacterial, fungal and protozoal infections that are difficult to control because of poor immunity.

### Answer 6
'Oligoclonal' antibodies are produced by more than one clone (family) of cells, but not by as many as are involved in the production of polyclonal

antibodies. 'Monoclonal' indicates that the antibodies are produced by a single clone of cells.

## Answer 7
Cell culture techniques of CD4 helper cells are available but we are unaware of their use in HIV-infected patients.

## Answer 8
In autoimmune disorders, the body generates immune responses against its own tissues, producing autoreactive T cells and autoantibodies. In normal development, T and B lymphocytes that recognize 'self' antigens are deleted in the thymus and bone marrow (central tolerance). Those that escape are suppressed by regulatory T cells in the circulation.

*Further reading*
*Clinical Medicine* (2006) July/Aug: 337–360 CME section on clinical immunology.

## Answer 9
1  Dexamethasone has very high glucocorticoid activity and therefore needs careful monitoring to avoid side-effects. Most trials on the use of corticosteroids have been performed with prednisolone, hence its common use.
2. All trials in MS are with methylprednisolone (1 g daily for 3 days), so it is better to use this agent.

## Answer 10
Yes; the pus cell is a neutrophil.

## Answer 11
Dendritic cells can change their expression of chemokine receptors and migrate from the mucosa to the lymph nodes. Dendritic cells are of several types and are similar to monocytes (myeloid dendritic cells), plasma cells (plasmacytoid) and follicular cells, which are probably not of haemopoeitic origin).

## Answer 12
1. Many advocate monthly monitoring, but on long-term azathioprine 3-monthly will often suffice.
2. Serum transferases: measurement of thiopurine methyltransferase (TPMT) levels before starting therapy can predict patients who will have a toxic reaction to azathioprine.

## Answer 13
We normally use a dose of 2 mg/kg and stick to it unless there are problems.

## QUESTIONS

**Question 1**
Please give examples of red meat, white meat and lean meat.

**Question 2**
What is lean body weight and how does it differ from routine measurement?

**Question 3**
Is the combination of drugs sibutramine and orlistat more effective in reducing obesity than using these on their own?

**Question 4**
Why does vitamin $B_{12}$ deficiency cause glossitis?

**Question 5**
Is a dosage of 2.5 mg/day of methyltestosterone, as a component in some multivitamin formulae, safe in the long-term?

**Question 6**
What is the effect of sodium/potassium imbalance on the microminerals?

**Question 7**
What is the role of fluoride in healing?

**Question 8**
In *K&C 6e (Box 5.6, p. 263)* it states 'Do not drink [alcohol] during the daytime'. Please explain why this is not recommended.

**Question 9**
Could you please tell me about the aetiology of 'refeeding syndrome'?

## Question 10
What is the Atkin's diet?

## Question 11
What is meant by bariatric surgical procedures?

## Question 12
In a patient with marked obesity, is bariatric surgery better than a balloon inserted into the stomach?

## Question 13
Does intravenous nutrition always have to be given via a central vein?

## Question 14
Why has there been an explosion of obesity in the young?

## Question 15
Are proteins mostly absorbed from the intestinal lumen into the blood as amino acids?

## Question 16
What are 'congeners' in alcohol?

## Question 17
Cholesterol is synthesized in the body. What is the comparative role of diet and endogenous production in the level of serum cholesterol?

## Question 18
We frequently read of the severe but 'rare' side-effect of myositis with statins. Do these drugs have more 'common' side-effects?

## Question 19
Is there a relationship between brain disease and alcohol intake? Does alcohol have a proven toxic effect on the brain?

## ANSWERS

**Answer 1**
- Red meat: beef, lamb.
- White meat: chicken, turkey.
- Lean meat: ostrich, venison.

**Answer 2**
Lean body mass approximates fat-free mass; it is not used in routine clinical nutrition. There is a formula for its calculation – if you really want it!

**Answer 3**
No; there is no additive effect and there is no interaction between the drugs.

**Answer 4**
Vitamin $B_{12}$ plays a major role in the formation of DNA (*see K&C 6e, Fig. 8.12, p. 431*). Many epithelial cells show evidence of atrophy, including the tongue – hence the glossitis, small bowel and stomach.

**Answer 5**
Yes, as far as anyone knows (see Chapter 19, Question 32).

**Answer 6**
We know of no evidence of sodium/potassium imbalance affecting microminerals.

**Answer 7**
Fluoride might stimulate new bone formation but this is of no clinical value. Fluoride is added to water to prevent dental caries.

**Answer 8**
'Do not drink during the daytime' is good advice in that it shortens the time available to drink and helps drinkers keep their consumption low. It is particularly useful advice to those who work in the wine and spirit trade.

**Answer 9**
The 'refeeding syndrome' occurs after feeding has restarted in severely malnourished patients. The features are:
- Fluid overload leading to heart failure sometimes producing acute pulmonary oedema. Sodium and water reabsorption in the kidney is increased by insulin, and the low serum albumin also contributes to the fluid overload.

- Hypokalaemia, hypomagnesaemia and hypophosphataemia occur as insulin stimulates cellular uptake of these ions.
- Cardiac arrhythmias are also prominent.

## Answer 10

The Atkins' diet is a low-carbohydrate diet used to promote weight loss. The principle is that the body will switch from burning glucose to burning fat. Atkins did (in addition to the diet) recommend exercise and nutritional supplements. However, like all diets, although there might be short-term gains, permanent weight loss is rare and patients should be encouraged to maintain the recommended healthy intake of food (Table 5.1).

## Answer 11

The term 'bariatric' is derived from a Greek word meaning 'weight'. Procedures are designed to reduce weight by restricting the size of the stomach or by passing the stomach. Stomach operations include:
- Gastric banding: a band is placed laparoscopically around the upper part of the stomach (lap-banding), creating a small pouch and a narrow passage into the stomach.

**Table 5.1 Recommended healthy dietary intake**

| Dietary component | Approximate amounts (% of total energy unless otherwise stated)* | General hints |
|---|---|---|
| Total carbohydrate | 55 (55–75) | Increase fruit, vegetables, beans, pasta, bread |
| Free sugar | 10 (<10) | Decrease sugary drinks |
| Protein | 15 (10–15) | Decrease red meat (see fat below) |
| Total fat | 30 (15–30) | Increase vegetable (including olive oil) and fish oil and decrease animal fat |
| Saturated fat | 10 (<10) | |
| Unsaturated fat | 20 | |
| Cholesterol | <300 (<300) mg/day | Decrease meat and eggs |
| Salt | <6 (<5) g/day | Decrease prepared meats and do not add extra salt to food |
| Total dietary fibre | 30 (>25) g/day | Increase fruit and vegetables and wholegrain foods |

*Values in parentheses are goals for the intake of populations, as given by the World Health Organization (including populations who are already on low-fat diets). Some of the extreme ranges are not realistic short-term goals for developed countries, e.g. 75% of total energy from carbohydrate and 15% fat. (From Kumar and Clarke Clinical Medicine 6e.)

- Vertical banded gastroplasty: a vertical band and staples create a small gastric pouch.

These are effective long-term treatments but have complications and side-effects.

## Answer 12
There are no comparative data as they are two different treatments. Balloon insertion into the stomach is used for 6 months only to help obese patients lose weight. Bariatric surgery (the favourite operation is lap-banding) is used on morbid obese patients when all medical therapy has failed.

## Answer 13
It is usual to give parenteral nutrition via a central catheter but there are specially formulated mixtures for use via a peripheral line. Peripheral parenteral nutrition is useful initially, as the catheter only lasts 5 days.

## Answer 14
There is no single lifestyle factor. There appear to be number of causes, including taking less exercise, watching television and playing computer games, as well as an increase in food intake, particularly of fatty, sugary foods that are very rich in calories. The different degrees of overweight are shown in Table 5.2.

## Answer 15
No, unlike carbohydrates, which are hydrolysed to monosaccharides and then absorbed, proteins are broken down to small peptides and only some amino acids prior to absorption.

## Answer 16
During the distillation process of spirits, in addition to ethyl alcohol, other alcohols (e.g. isoamyl alcohol) are produced. It is thought that these 'congeners' play a big role in 'hangovers'! Port and bourbon have a higher congener content than gin and vodka. Obviously, the quantity drunk also plays a role!

**Table 5.2** Ranges of body mass index (BMI) used to classify degrees of overweight and associated risk of comorbidities

| WHO classification | BMI (kg/m$^2$) | Risk of comorbidities |
|---|---|---|
| Overweight | 25–30 | Mildly increased |
| Obese | >30 | |
|    Class I | 30–35 | Moderate |
|    Class II | 35–40 | Severe |
|    Class III | > 40 | Very severe |

## Answer 17

Cholesterol is synthesized in the body, mainly in the liver. The higher the amount of cholesterol in the diet, the lower the amount of cholesterol synthesized, and vice versa. Thus, it is difficult to significantly lower your serum cholesterol by diet alone unless the diet is very restrictive. Familial hypercholesterolaemia is related to a reduction in the number of low-density lipoprotein (LDL) receptors.

## Answer 18

Gastrointestinal side-effects, including abdominal pain, flatulence, constipation, diarrhoea, nausea and vomiting, occur frequently but are often tolerated without complaint.

## Answer 19

Yes, alcohol has a toxic effect on the brain; try mental arithmetic after a few drinks. Alcohol causes blackouts and memory lapses, even in small amounts. Wernicke–Korsakoff syndrome due to thiamine deficiency is seen in chronic abusers, as are epilepsy and dementia.

# Gastrointestinal disease 6

## Question 1
Please explain the role of the sympathetic nervous system in the gastrointestinal tract.

## Question 2
What is the difference between a submandibular salivary gland swelling and swelling of a salivary lymph node?

## Question 3
How does Barrett's oesophagus develop?

## Question 4
Is it recommended to treat asymptomatic endoscopically diagnosed reflux oesophagitis with acid suppression and/or antireflux measures?

## Question 5
Is it recommended to give a young patient, diagnosed endoscopically to have mild reflux oesophagitis, life-long proton pump inhibitors (PPIs) to prevent the development of Barrett's oesophagitis?

## Question 6
Is it safe to give a patient with reflux oesophagitis who is on proton pump inhibitors (PPIs) for treatment of acid suppression, aspirin in antiplatelet doses (75–325 mg per day)?

## Question 7
Does a combination of magnesium and aluminium hydroxide salts, taken as antacid for reflux oesophagitis, have serious long-term adverse effects?

### Question 8
In the treatment of reflux oesophagitis with a proton pump inhibitor (PPI), should the PPI be life long or given for 4–8 weeks, as mentioned by the drug manufacturers?

### Question 9
Would a patient who suffers with reflux oesophagitis as a result of a hiatus hernia, and who is not responsive to proton pump inhibitors (PPIs), benefit from a highly selective vagotomy?

### Question 10
1. What are the causes of belching and what appropriate drug can be used?
2. What are the effects of smoking on the gastrointestinal tract and what is its role in peptic ulcer disease?

### Question 11
Dear authors, why are gastric ulcers more common along the lesser curve, near the pylorus of the stomach?

### Question 12
What is the best time of day to administer omeprazole, and why?

### Question 13
Is it safe to use the drugs omeprazole and ranitidine during pregnancy?

### Question 14
Are non-steroidal anti-inflammatory drugs harmful to the stomach when taken parenterally, for example by intravenous or intramuscular routes?

### Question 15
Is it safe to give a patient with a past history of bleeding peptic ulcer aspirin in an antiplatelet dose of 75–325 mg?

### Question 16
Is sulpiride effective in the treatment of a peptic ulcer or gastro-oesophageal reflux disease (GORD)?

### Question 17
Is clopidogrel gentle on the stomach?

### Question 18
Is there a drug interaction between non-steroidal anti-inflammatory drugs (NSAIDs) and proton pump inhibitors (PPIs)?

## Question 19
Do antacids enhance mucosal resistance in the gastric mucosa? If so, please indicate the mechanism.

## Question 20
Is there a drug interaction between antacids and $H_2$-receptor blockers?

## Question 21
Does the combination of aluminium and magnesium hydroxide, given as an antacid, decrease the absorption of omeprazole if these are co-administered to help relieve heartburn quickly?

## Question 22
Should proton pump inhibitors be used with caution in patients with renal impairment?

## Question 23
Has cisapride been withdrawn from the market because of the danger of ventricular fibrillation?

## Question 24
In peptic ulcer disease:
1. What are the indications for an upper gastrointestinal endoscopy?
2. As this is an invasive procedure, is an oesophagogastroduodenoscopy (OGD) or barium meal X-ray preferable?

## Question 25
Is telithromycin as, or more, effective than clarithromycin in the treatment of *Helicobacter pylori*? If so, what is the recommended dosage and how long should treatment be continued?

## Question 26
Currently favoured regimens for eradication of *Helicobacter pylori* are triple therapy with a proton pump inhibitor along with two antibiotics for 1 week. For example:
- Omeprazole 20 mg + metronidazole 400 mg and clarithromycin 500 mg (all twice daily).
- Omeprazole 20 mg + clarithromycin 500 mg and amoxicillin 1 g (all twice daily).

Resistance to amoxicillin has not yet been demonstrated.

Previously, regimens such as omeprazole, metronidazole, amoxicillin and clarithromycin were recommended; are these regimens no longer used? The reason behind this question is the 'sky-high' cost of clarithromycin in Pakistan, which is inversely proportional to patient compliance (that is, low-cost regimens tend to have a higher rate of compliance).

## Question 27

What is the difference between the management of a gastric and of a duodenal ulcer?

## Question 28

How does omeprazole suppress *Helicobacter pylori*?

## Question 29

Does omeprazole cause rebound hyperacidity? Does this also apply to $H_2$-blockers?

## Question 30

On (*K&C 6e, p.273*), you state that the postsynaptic neurotransmitter that inhibits the relaxation of lower oesophageal sphincter (LOS) is nitric oxide (NO). I have understood NO to promote relaxation of LOS by acting on the non-adrenergic, non-cholinergic (NANC) inhibitory neurones, which inhibits the action of cholinergic excitatory neurones. Could you please explain this paradox?

## Question 31

It is stated that nitric oxide (NO) inhibits the relaxation of the lower oesophageal sphincter (LOS) and that sildenafil is given for treating achalasia. As far as I know, sildenafil acts to increase the guanine monophosphate (GMP), just as NO uses the same mechanism to relax the LOS. Could you explain this paradox?

## Question 32

In Kumar and Clark *Clinical Medicine* you mention that auscultation is not important in cases of gastrointestinal disorders, but Harrison's *Principles of Internal Medicine* gives this as being of equal importance because succussion splash and bowel sounds can help in presumptive diagnosis. Succussion splash indicates gastric obstruction (e.g. gastroparesis) and likewise bowel sounds can help determine the status of developing ileus. Would you agree that this is therefore a diagnostic tool?

## Question 33

Is it hazardous to give aspirin in the antiplatelet doses (75–325 mg/day) to a patient with a past history of haematemesis proved to be from a peptic ulcer?

## Question 34

How can upper gastrointestinal (GI) bleeding be distinguished from lower GI bleeding by using faecal analysis?

## Question 35

In upper gastrointestinal bleeding, without knowing the cause or source of bleeding, why do we give proton pump inhibitors (PPIs, e.g. omeprazole)? What is the role of these, if the source of bleeding is not peptic or duodenal ulcer?

## Question 36

Why is the incidence of coeliac disease increasing in many countries?

## Question 37

Are small amounts of gluten harmful to a patient with coeliac disease?

## Question 38

I refer to the treatment of complications related to diverticular disease. Under 'bleeding' you mention that 'Persistent bleeding can often be arrested by undertaking an "instant" barium enema, which acts to plug the offending diverticulum'. When I mentioned this to my consultant he said he had never heard of this. Could you clarify how this would work and where I could obtain more information?

## Question 39

In children with abdominal pain and fever, does a white cell count help establish a diagnosis of appendicitis?

## Question 40

I have always been taught that ulcerative colitis only affects the large bowel with some associated proctitis. I read in your chapter on gastrointestinal disease that it can cause mouth ulcers and am now confused.

## Question 41

In pseudomembranous colitis, what is the first treatment of choice, metronidazole or vancomycin?

## Question 42

Is Crohn's disease considered as an autoimmune disease. If it is, are there other predisposing factors to it other than genetics? If it is not, what is its nature?

## Question 43

Why does carcinoma of the ascending colon cause more anaemia than obstruction, and carcinoma of the descending colon more obstruction features and less anaemia?

## Question 44
Can you explain why a patient with colorectal carcinoma might present with diarrhoea and abdominal pain?

## Question 45
What causes the blood to be altered in the presentation of melaena: is it intestinal juice?

## Question 46
What is the differential diagnosis of multiple rectal ulcers in an 18-year-old female?

## Question 47
What is the best surgical technique in a chronic (2–3 years) painful anal fissure that is located sagittally posteriorly?

## Question 48
Can I make a diagnosis of irritable bowel syndrome (IBS) in a 40-year-old female patient without doing gastrointestinal investigations?

## Question 49
What is the cause of abdominal bloating, which is often a symptom in patients with irritable bowel syndrome (IBS)?

## Question 50
1. Where is the Traub's area situated anatomically?
2. What does it mean if it is dull on percussion?
3. What is the proper way to percuss this area?

## Question 51
In general, it is claimed that only water and some salts are absorbed in the large gut, whereas the small gut is practically free of bacteria (which are present only in the large gut). In a patient on broad-spectrum antibiotics, bleeding can occur as a result of vitamin K deficiency. If the flora synthesizing vitamin K is disturbed, how can vitamin deficiency occur when the large gut is not supposed to absorb? How can this be due to a change in bacterial flora?

## ANSWERS

### Answer 1
Sympathetic fibres are distributed along the entire length of the gut; the stimulation or inhibition of these plays a role in many aspects of gut motility. Increased sympathetic stimulation produces the well-known anxiety symptoms, for example before exams when increased stimulation produces diarrhoea.

### Answer 2
The salivary lymph glands are part of the superficial lymphatic drainage of the neck; enlargement occurs in infection and in malignant disease. The submandibular gland is swollen if there is blockage of the duct or if a tumour is present. It can also be affected by the mumps virus, although parotid involvement is more common.

### Answer 3
Barrett's oesophagus is defined as areas of columnar epithelium with intestinal metaplasia extending upwards in the lower oesophagus replacing the normal squamous epithelium. It is due to chronic gastro-oesophageal reflux.

### Answer 4
No, it is not recommended to treat asymptomatic reflux oesophagitis. However, many gastroenterologists *do* treat it in the hope that long-term complications (e.g. stricture, Barrett's and cancer) can be averted.

### Answer 5
No, there is no indication to give long-term PPIs in patients with mild reflux oesophagitis; there is no evidence that this prevents the development of Barrett's.

### Answer 6
Yes, it is safe to give aspirin to a patient already on a PPI, which is – of course – cytoprotective.

### Answer 7
No, there are no serious long-term adverse effects. Usually, however, in patients who require long-term treatment, an $H_2$-receptor antagonist or a proton pump inhibitor is used.

### Answer 8
Patients with reflux oesophagitis usually have a low lower oesophageal sphincter pressure, so that reflux is a permanent event. After stopping

PPIs, the symptoms return and life-long therapy may be necessary. Some would regard this as an indication for surgery.

### Answer 9
No. A highly selective vagotomy will only do the same as the PPIs, that is, reduce the acid output. Try increasing the dose of the PPI to twice daily.

### Answer 10
1. Belching is due to swallowing air. It is often picked up as a habit and it is not usually associated with pathology. Occasionally, patients who have upper gastrointestinal symptoms, such as heartburn or abdominal discomfort, swallow air in an attempt to ease their symptoms, and end up belching. Treatment can be difficult; no drugs are effective.
2. Smoking impairs the healing of peptic ulcer disease and also makes gastro-oesophageal reflux worse. It is also associated with relapse in patients with Crohn's disease (but not in ulcerative colitis) but nevertheless therefore all patients with Crohn's should be encouraged to stop smoking.

### Answer 11
There is no definitive reason why gastric ulcers are more common on the lesser curve. They are usually just distal to the transitional zone between the body (acid-secreting mucosa) and antrum (non-acid-secreting mucosa). Reflux of bile and other duodenal contents into the stomach is thought to play a role.

### Answer 12
Either morning or evening. It has a prolonged action so that the effect lasts over 24 hours.

### Answer 13
Neither drug is recommended in pregnancy, but ranitidine is probably safe. No drug should be used in pregnancy unless absolutely essential.

### Answer 14
Yes; the inhibition of gastric mucosal cyclo-oxygenase (COX) activity is a systemic effect.

### Answer 15
A patient with a bleeding peptic ulcer, which is usually due to *Helicobacter pylori*, should have eradication therapy. In the case of a bleeding ulcer, eradication must be checked with a $^{13}$C urea breath test or a stool antigen test. When eradication has been shown to be successful, it

is safe to use low-dose aspirin. (*Note*: patients with and without a history of ulcers can bleed even with low-dose aspirin.)

### Answer 16
Sulpiride is not used. It does have an antimuscarinic action, which would reduce acid production, but in GORD this is offset by a reduction in lower oesophageal sphincter tone. It is therefore not useful in peptic ulcer or GORD.

### Answer 17
Clopidogrel does cause dyspepsia and abdominal pain, and it can lead to gastrointestinal bleeding. So, is it 'gentle'? The answer must be 'No'.

### Answer 18
There is no drug interaction. Indeed, PPIs are used as mucosal cytoprotective agents in patients on NSAIDs.

### Answer 19
If, by antacids, you mean aluminium hydroxide or magnesium trisilicate the answer is 'Yes', but only in very large doses. They work by neutralizing acid, which in turn makes the mucosa more resistant to damage. A proton pump inhibitor is more practical.

### Answer 20
No, but there is little point in using both except for immediate symptom relief, e.g. with an alginate containing antacid in gastro-oesophageal reflux disease (GORD).

### Answer 21
Omeprazole is formulated as enteric-coated granules and is absorbed in the small intestine. Antacids therefore have no effect on its absorption.

### Answer 22
No.

### Answer 23
Yes, it increases the Q-Tc interval.

### Answer 24
1. Endoscopy is used in:
   - Gastric ulcer: for diagnosis and to take biopsies to exclude malignancy; it is also used for follow-up of gastric ulcers.
   - Duodenal ulcer: for diagnosis, although in young patients with *Helicobacter pylori* antibodies and typical history endoscopy is not necessary.

2. Good double-contrast barium meals are comparable to endoscopy but as biopsies cannot be taken (e.g. for *H. pylori* and malignancy), their use is becoming less frequent.

## Answer 25

Telithromycin is a newly introduced macrolide and should be effective in *H. pylori* eradication regimens, 800 mg × 2 daily. However, you are always better to stick to the tried and tested – in this case the macrolide clarithromycin – until the evidence changes.

## Answer 26

The problem is metronidazole resistance, which runs at 50% at least and is probably higher in some areas. The other problem is the cost, as you say. It might be reasonable in your country to try omeprazole, metronidazole, amoxicillin and use clarithromycin instead of metronidazole for treatment failures. Tetracycline has been used in combination regimens it is also cheap and is a possible alternative to clarithromycin.

## Answer 27

Most duodenal ulcers and 80% of gastric ulcers are due to *Helicobacter pylori* infection. Eradication therapy of the organism is the same. It is usual to check that a gastric ulcer has healed (thereby excluding a malignant ulcer) by doing repeat gastroscopy; this is not necessary for duodenal ulcers.

## Answer 28

*In vitro*, omeprazole inhibits the growth of *H. pylori* below pH 7. Clinically, it is thought that omeprazole enhances the local immune response by increasing intragastric pH. It also reduces the washout of antibiotics from the mucosa and lowers the inhibitory concentrations of pH-sensitive antibiotics.

## Answer 29

Rebound increased acid secretion lasting about 2 months occurs after 40 mg a day of omeprazole for 2 days. Yes, rebound hyperacidity also occurs after withdrawing histamine $H_2$-receptor antagonists.

## Answer 30

The LOS is tonically closed at rest. This resting tone is maintained by both myogenic properties and active tonic neural excitation. The reduction in tone and reduction of the LOS that occurs with swallowing is under the control of cholinergic and NANC neurones. As you say, NO acts on the NANC inhibitory neurones, which inhibit the excitatory cholinergic neurones, thus reducing acetylcholine release.

## Answer 31

In achalasia there is a selective loss of the inhibitory neurones in the myenteric plexus. This leads to excitation of the smooth muscle at the LOS by mediators such as acetylcholine. Sildenafil increases NO production. It is the NO-containing neurones that are particularly affected in achalasia so that relaxation of the sphincter is impaired.

## Answer 32

In practice, outside the emergency room or postoperatively (looking for ileus), bowel sounds are not helpful. A succussion splash can indicate gastric obstruction but is seldom helpful in practice.

## Answer 33

Any patient who has bled from a peptic ulcer – and who is therefore presumably *Helicobacter pylori* (HP) positive – should have eradication therapy. Successful eradication of HP following a bleed must be checked with either an HP breath test or a stool test. After eradication, the same risks of aspirin therapy apply as to the normal population.

## Answer 34

There are no reliable ways of distinguishing lower from upper gastrointestinal bleeding by faecal analysis. Obviously bright red blood suggests lower GI bleeding – except when blood loss is huge, when blood loss from higher up can be bright red blood. Altered blood, e.g. a melaena stool, is from lesions proximal to the caecum.

## Answer 35

Approximately 50% of cases of GI bleeding are from peptic ulcer disease, and a PPI (e.g. omeprazole) reduces the rate of recurrent bleeding and the need for surgery. In many patients it is initially unclear where the bleeding is coming from, so PPIs tend to be given to everybody even though they have never been shown to be of value in, for example, variceal bleeding.

## Answer 36

The answer is that we have better serological screening tests, e.g. tissue transglutaminase and endomysial antibodies, which are now being used extensively. The general awareness of coeliac disease has also increased.

## Answer 37

Theoretically, yes! However, even a gluten-free diet has very tiny amounts of gluten and probably these small amounts are not overtly harmful in most patients. A few patients might be very sensitive.

## Answer 38

This is anecdotal data and is probably incorrect; often the bleeding stops spontaneously. We have decided to remove this anecdotal piece of advice from the 6th edition.

## Answer 39

Between 70 and 90% of patients with appendicitis have a raised white cell count >15000. This has a sensitivity of 20–60%, with a specificity of 85–100% in children with appendicitis. Imaging (e.g. ultrasound and computed tomography) should now be used to make a diagnosis of appendicitis.

## Answer 40

You have been correctly taught. Ulcerative colitis (UC) only affects the large bowel, i.e. the colon and rectum, with a small number of patients having some inflammation of the very distal part of the ileum (called backwash ileitis). This distinguishes UC from Crohn's disease, which affects anywhere from the mouth to the anus, most commonly the small and large bowel. Both diseases are, however, associated with 'non-specific' mouth ulcers, which also occur in a number of gastrointestinal diseases (e.g. coeliac disease) and other conditions (e.g. Behçet's disease).

## Answer 41

Metronidazole is the first choice, largely due to the cost of oral vancomycin.

## Answer 42

Crohn's disease is not usually considered to be an autoimmune disease, although the immune system is very involved in the pathological process. We do not know the exact cause of Crohn's disease but it is felt by most that some aetiological agent (perhaps a bacterium?) stimulates the immune system to over-respond in a genetically susceptible person. *CARD 15* gene mutations contribute to disease susceptibility.

*Further reading*
Podolsky D (2002) Inflammatory bowel disease. *New England Journal of Medicine* **347**: 417–429.

## Answer 43

Carcinoma of the caecum and ascending colon tend to bleed and cause anaemia but not obstruction because of the large size and 'give' in the right side of the colon. The reverse is true of the descending colon; a carcinoma is more likely to obstruct the smaller, more rigid left colon.

## Answer 44

Very often, the symptoms are not related and the colorectal cancer is found incidentally when a patient is investigated for pain or diarrhoea.

Right-sided colonic lesions do not usually produce gut symptoms. Lesions in the sigmoid do, probably by partial obstruction.

## Answer 45
No; it is bacteria.

## Answer 46
Multiple rectal ulcers are common in inflammatory bowel disease. They also occur in infective proctitis (e.g. due to amoebae) or in sexually transmitted infections (e.g. herpes viral infections). Rectal spread occurs in gonococcal infection and can produce ulcers. The answer is to take samples for cultures and biopsies for histological diagnosis.

## Answer 47
A lateral internal sphincterotomy is the best surgical procedure. This is the advice of the American Gastroenterological Association (AGA) in its Medical Position Statement 2002.

## Answer 48
You must first make sure that there are no 'alarm' symptoms (Box 6.1). Take a very careful history because most patients of this age with IBS will have a preceding history of IBS. Simple blood tests and a follow-up of the patient are also very helpful in the diagnosis.

## Answer 49
This is difficult to answer! We agree this is a very common symptom. It is not due to air/wind, which most patients think.

## Answer 50
Traub's space is an area of resonance overlying the gas bubble in the left lateral hemithorax. Its size and localization depend on the contents and position of the stomach. Percuss with the patient on his or her right side.

## Answer 51
Small amounts of menaquinones (a form of vitamin K), which are synthesized by bacteria, are absorbed in the colon.

---

**Box 6.1** Alarm symptoms: indications for upper gastrointestinal endoscopy

- Dysphagia
- Weight loss
- Protracted vomiting
- Anorexia
- Haematemesis or malaena

# 7 Liver, biliary tract and pancreatic disease

**Question 1**
Please could you tell me the normal range of values for the liver function test serum alkaline phosphatase. The only mention of the parameters is that a reading of >1000 = serious liver condition.

**Question 2**
What is the best single test of liver function to exclude liver cell failure in the routine work-up of a patient with early dementia?

**Question 3**
How valuable is the measurement of the liver span in a physical examination?

**Question 4**
Why has the term 'chronic liver disease' replaced terms such as 'chronic hepatitis'? What exactly does this new term mean and what conditions does it cover?

**Question 5**
Can jaundice occur early in schistosomal hepatic fibrosis and, if so, how?

**Question 6**
My patient has been found to have a serum bilirubin of 34 μmol/L (2 mg/dL) on three occasions. The other liver tests are normal. He tells me he has Gilbert's disease; how can I prove this?

**Question 7**
Why is urinary urobilinogen increased in haemolytic jaundice? If the bilirubin in this condition is unconjugated, how does it reach the terminal ileum to be converted into urobilinogen?

## Question 8
How does cholestatic jaundice affect the kidney?

## Question 9
What is the mechanism by which cholestatic jaundice causes bradycardia?

## Question 10
Are 'jaundice' and 'icterus' one and the same? I was taught that icterus is yellowing of the sclera, while jaundice is yellowing of the skin and the mucous membranes. As a result, carotenaemia can produce jaundice but not icterus: is this so? I would be grateful if you would clarify this for me.

## Question 11
I am a third-year student nurse and am currently researching a case study based on the biopsychosocial history of a patient who suffers from chronic hepatitis C, which initially occurred as a result of injecting drugs. I am confused about the biological effect of hepatitis: how exactly does it affect the liver?

## Question 12
What are the admission criteria for a case of acute viral hepatitis?

## Question 13
I would like to know where I can find details on hepatitis B virus (HBV) infection: chronic carrier, asymptomatic [normal liver function tests, HBV DNA/real-time polymerase chain reaction (PCR) = 240 copies/mL, core less than 0.1]. Does a patient with such a profile need therapy or fine needle aspiration (FNA) biopsy? What is the possibility of hepatocellular carcinoma (HCC) in such a patient?

## Question 14
In chronic hepatitis B virus (HBV) infection, when anti-hepatitis B e antibody (anti-HBe) develops (seroconversion), the antigen disappears and there is a rise in alanine transferase (ALT). However, the graph in your book (K&C 6e, p. 365, Fig. 7.16) seems to show a fall in ALT at this point. Which is correct?

## Question 15
Interferon can be used in prophylaxis from hepatitis C after exposure. Could you explain how this can be used, and what degree of success can be expected as a result?

## Question 16
What is the latest recommended drug treatment for hepatitis C?

## Question 17
Can hepatitis C disease be treated in a carrier state completely by giving interferon?

## Question 18
I am a carrier of hepatitis C (HCV) and am going to have antiviral treatment soon. Are the side-effects of antiviral treatment for HCV bound to occur? I am very worried.

## Question 19
Besides needle-pricks, how else is it possible to contract hepatitis C from a hepatitis C (HCV)-positive patient? Are the patient's skin/sweat (or other bodily secretions) infectious?

## Question 20
What is the risk of infection with hepatitis C from blood splashed into the eyes?

## Question 21
Hepatitis C (HCV): if results from the polymerase chain reaction (PCR) examination are inconclusive, what does this mean? Should further investigations be undertaken and, if so, will there be a risk of chronicity?

## Question 22
In a patient with hepatitis C and autoimmune hepatitis, can corticosteroids be prescribed for the autoimmune hepatitis?

## Question 23
We were told that the more vascular a structure is, the more antigen (HLA/blood groups) matching is needed for transplantation, e.g. cornea transplant needs no matching. However, the liver is a very vascular organ; I don't know why liver transplantation needs blood group matching only but renal transplantation needs much more HLA matching.

## Question 24
About steatohepatitis: please give me more information about the occurrence of cirrhosis in such patients (non-alcoholic) and is there any role and indication for lipotropic agents and hypocholesterolaemic drugs?

## Question 25
I am working on non-alcoholic fatty liver disease (NAFLD) but I did not find anything regarding it. Can you tell me about its relationship with lipids?

## Question 26
Is NASH a valid term or not and what manifestation has it?

## Question 27
Is terlipressin better in controlling variceal bleeding than somatostatin?

## Question 28
Why is there a hyperdynamic circulation in cirrhosis?

## Question 29
Why is there an increased level of immunoglobulin G (IgG) in patients with cirrhosis?

## Question 30
Cirrhosis of liver is reversible according to your book. What is the progress and when will we be able to counteract the 'tissue inhibitors of metalloproteinases' (TIMPs) and thus save the lives of our patients?

## Question 31
What are the criteria for knowing the prognosis of cirrhosis (Child's criteria)?

## Question 32
What is the recommended treatment for cirrhosis of the liver?

## Question 33
Is there any role for liver dialysis in hepatic encephalopathy?

## Question 34
I have been asked to write an essay on 'caring' for a client who has been an alcohol abuser for more than 10 years and is in the 'recovery' stage. I am aware there are many different factors, such as length of abuse, amount consumed, age, gender etc. . . . My question is: how long will it take the liver to 'recover' or to return to normal after stopping drinking? I am especially interested in blood tests, fatty deposits and gamma-glutamyl transpeptidases ($\gamma$-GTs).

## Question 35
Can patients with liver cell failure suffer from myocardial infarction?

## Question 36
What is the definition of liver cell failure (decompensated liver disease?

### Question 37

Flapping tremors: why do we get flapping tremors and no other types of tremor in liver failure? What is their mechanism and in which other conditions do they occur?

### Question 38

In a patient with liver cell failure, can there be resting and action tremors or parkinsonian features if it is confirmed that the patient does not have Wilson's disease?

### Question 39

Does the absence of any cirrhosis of the liver, together with normal liver enzymes, in a 9-year-old boy complaining of chorea of a 5-year duration, exclude Wilson's disease?

### Question 40

Can Wilson's disease be excluded in a patient complaining of movement disorder for over 2 years, when there is an absence of cirrhotic liver change?

### Question 41

What drugs cause Budd–Chiari syndrome?

### Question 42

I recently saw a patient with pyrexia of unknown origin (PUO). He was not particularly unwell and not jaundiced. But 1 week later he was found to have a liver abscess on ultrasound. How can one make the diagnosis earlier?

### Question 43

What is the most recent management of HCC (hepatocellular carcinoma)? What is radiofrequency ablation? What is its role in the management of HCC and its prognosis?

### Question 44

How do you differentiate haemorrhagic ascitic fluid due to malignancy and accidental rupture of blood vessel while withdrawing the fluid?

### Question 45

Is there any place for the medical treatment of gallstones with ursodeoxycholic acid?

### Question 46

In a case of common bile duct stones, where it is acknowledged that spontaneous passage within 24 hours is observed in approximately 50% of patients provided the stone is small, and that in these cases there is no need for a sphincterotomy, is the use of antispasmodics, e.g. Buscopan (active ingredient hyoscine-N-butylbromide), recommended? Surely these will reduce the pain and improve the chance of a spontaneous release of obstruction without surgical procedure?

## Question 47
What is sphincter of Oddi dysfunction?

## Question 48
I would like to know: what is the role of lysosomal hydrolases (cathepsin B) in the pathogenesis of acute pancreatitis?

## Question 49
What is the role of octreotide in management of acute pancreatitis?

## Question 50
Why does paralytic ileus occur in pancreatitis?

## Question 51
How sensitive is the increase in serum lipase levels in the case of acute pancreatitis?

## Question 52
What is the association between chronic pancreatitis and peripheral vascular disease (PVD)?

## Question 53
Please, can you explain to us the mechanism of pancreatitis in hypertriglyceridaemias?

## Question 54
Is there any role for chemotherapy in carcinoma of the pancreas?

## Question 55
1. How should portal hypertension be managed in patients with bronchial asthma, where beta-blockers are contraindicated?
2. How should diuretics for these patients with hypertension be added?

## Question 56
Is cirrhosis a prerequisite for the development of hepatocellular carcinoma (HCC) in hepatitis B (HBV)?

## Question 57
Should therapy with interferons in the treatment of hepatitis C (HCV) and hepatitis B (HBV) commence when the polymerase chain reaction (PCR) is positive, irrespective of serum glutamyl pyruvate transaminase (SGPT) levels?

## ANSWERS

### Answer 1
The normal serum alkaline phosphatase is 40–100 IU/L. Levels of 400+ are common in cholestatic liver disease. Levels of 1000 and over are seen in primary biliary cirrhosis and liver metastases. (*Note*: remember alkaline phosphatase is also found in bone so that bone disease, e.g. Paget's, is also associated with a raised serum alkaline phosphatase.)

### Answer 2
Liver function is assessed with the serum albumin as the well as the prothrombin time. The other routine liver tests, e.g. transferases and alkaline phosphatase reflect liver damage not function. You can therefore measure either the prothrombin time or the albumin.

### Answer 3
Quite useful but less valuable since the widespread use of ultrasound scans.

### Answer 4
Chronic liver disease is a general term for all types of liver disease that are chronic (by definition greater than 6 months' duration). It has not replaced terms such as chronic hepatitis, which is used for a hepatitis that is chronic.

### Answer 5
No. Hepatocellular function remains good.

### Answer 6
In Gilbert's, hepatic glucuronidation of bilirubin is 30% of normal so that there is excess of unconjugated bilirubin. To prove the diagnosis you should measure the total and unconjugated bilirubin in the serum, the unconjugated will be high. A normal reticulocyte count will exclude haemolysis and you have the diagnosis. Genetic studies are not necessary.

### Answer 7
This is because increased unconjugated bilirubin also leads to some increase in conjugated bilirubin, which can then be secreted into the gut and converted to urobilinogen.

### Answer 8
Cholestatic jaundice does produce tubular necrosis, albeit rarely. This can occur following surgery. It can be prevented by intravenous infusion of mannitol.

## Answer 9
It used to be said that this was due to the effect of the high level of bile salts on the sinoatrial node. However, recent evidence suggests that bradycardia in adults is rare in cholestatic jaundice.

## Answer 10
'Jaundice' and 'icterus' are the same. In the main, people use the word 'jaundice' most of the time. 'Anicteric' is sometimes used to describe a person who is not jaundiced.

## Answer 11
Hepatitis means inflammation of the liver. It can occur from many causes but in your patient the hepatitis C virus seems to have been the cause of the inflammation. 60–80% of patients who develop hepatitis C go on to chronic liver disease; 20–30% of these will develop cirrhosis of the liver over a period of 20–30 years. The damage to the liver in the chronic situation is due to the immunological response to the hepatitis C virus.

## Answer 12
Most patients with acute viral hepatitis do not need to be admitted to hospital. Patients who appear to be developing hepatic failure do need admission. Clinical features are then of a severely jaundiced patient with some degree of drowsiness.

## Answer 13
The patient described is sometimes referred to as a 'healthy carrier'. These patients seem tolerant of the virus and the prognosis is very good.

Liver histology in such patients shows no significant damage and biopsies or therapy are not recommended.

90% of patients who are HBV carriers who develop HCC have cirrhosis, which is rare in a healthy carrier as described above.

### Further reading
Lok AS, Heathcote EJ, Hoofnagle JH (2001) Management of hepatitis B. *Gastroenterology* **120**: 1828–1853. Online. Available: http://www.hepb.org/NIH.html

## Answer 14
When seroconversion occurs there may be a 'flare', i.e. a short rise in ALT, but then the ALT falls usually to normal. This is reflected in the graph.

## Answer 15
Monotherapy with 5 M units daily for 4 weeks then 5 M units three times a week for 20 weeks of alpha-interferon was used in one trial with a high

success rate, (i.e. no RNA detected). Pegylated interferon can probably be used instead; there are no trials as yet.

## Answer 16

Pegylated interferon combined with ribavirin. The dosage and length of treatment depends on the genotype.

*Further reading*
Hoofnagle JH, Seoff LB (2006) Peg interferon and ribavirin for chronic hepatitis C. *New England Journal of Medicine* **355**: 2444–2451.

## Answer 17

There is strictly no carrier state for hepatitis C because there is always some degree of liver damage in patients who have persistence of the virus.

At the present time, the treatment of hepatitis C is pegylated interferon and ribavirin. Treatment should be given to those patients with chronic hepatitis on liver histology, HCV RNA in their serum and who have had raised serum aminotransferases for more than 6 months. Patients who have persistently *normal* aminotransferases and abnormal histology can also be treated with the same combination.

## Answer 18

Some side-effects are almost universal with interferon, although pegylated interferon produces fewer side-effects. You must discuss the treatment with your specialist.

## Answer 19

Only blood spread is implicated in HCV hepatitis. Sexual spread is rare.

## Answer 20

It is rare. There is only one reported case.

## Answer 21

PCR testing for HCV RNA is very variable, depending on the laboratory used and on the technique. In addition, the HCV RNA may only be present in small amounts and viraemia may be intermittent. Repeat tests at 6 months.

## Answer 22

Yes, under careful supervision. Treatment of the hepatitis C should also be undertaken if treatment criteria are met.

## Answer 23

The liver is a vascular organ that often behaves as a 'privileged tissue' in that little immune reaction occurs. The liver appears to induce a state of suppression by the secretion of large amounts of donor-soluble major histocompatibility (MHC) class 1 antigen with the migration of large numbers of donor dendritic cells from the donor liver into the host. This was first shown by Sir Roy Calne in pigs.

## Answer 24

Non-alcoholic steatohepatitis (NASH) is now thought to be a subgroup of patients with non-alcoholic fatty liver disease (NAFLD). With NASH, not only is there fat in the liver but there is inflammation on liver histology obtained at biopsy.

Cirrhosis does occur in patients with NASH, so that liver biopsies are probably indicated in patients with NAFLD and raised transferases (over 100 IU).

Weight reduction, drugs to lower cholesterol and triglycerides are used but there is no good evidence of their efficacy.

*Further reading*

Maher J (2001) Antidiabetic treatment for NASH. *Hepatology* **33**: 1338–1339.
Teli MR, James OF, Burt AD et al. (1995) The natural history of nonalcoholic fatty liver: a follow-up study. *Hepatology* **22**: 1714–1719.

## Answer 25

It has been recognized for many years that a fatty liver is sometimes found in patients who do not drink alcohol. The term 'non-alcoholic steatohepatitis' (NASH) was introduced in the 1990s. Subsequently, it has been recognized that some patients have a fatty liver on biopsy with no accompanying inflammation; this group is called non-alcoholic fatty liver disease (NAFLD). It seems that only patients with evidence of NASH on biopsy progress to chronic liver disease with fibrosis and cirrhosis. Some of these patients do have high lipid levels (both cholesterol and triglycerides) but this is by no means invariable. NAFLD is associated with the metabolic syndrome (Box 7.1).

---

### Box 7.1  Metabolic syndrome (NCEP APT III*)

Three or more of the following:
- High blood pressure (>130/85 mmHg)
- Elevated serum triglycerides (>150 mg/dL or 1.695 mmol/L)
- Decreased HDL cholesterol (<40 mg/dL or <0.9 mmol/L in men and <50 mg/dL or <1 mmol/L in women)
- Increased abdominal circumference [>102 cm (40 inches) men or >88 cm (35 inches) women]
- Impaired fasting glucose (>110 mg/dL or >6.1 mmol/L)

\* National Cholesterol Education Programme Adult Treatment Panel III

*Further reading*
Malnick SD et al (2003) Nonalcoholic fatty liver disease. *Quarterly Journal of Medicine* **96**: 699–709.
National Cholesterol Education Adult Treatment Programme III (2001) *Journal of the American Medical Association* **285**: 2486–2497.

## Answer 26

NASH, non-alcoholic steatohepatitis, was introduced a few years ago for patients with fatty liver not due to alcohol. The meaning has now been changed slightly in that the term 'NASH' is used only for a small group of patients with non-alcoholic fatty liver (NAFL) who have inflammation as well as fat on liver histology.

*Further reading*
Malnick SD et al (2003) Nonalcoholic fatty liver disease. *Quarterly Journal of Medicine* **96**: 699–709.

## Answer 27

Terlipressin has been shown to reduce mortality but has more side-effects than somatostatin.

## Answer 28

The hyperdynamic circulation that occurs is partly due to the opening of portosystemic collaterals. In addition, there are increased levels of circulatory vasodilators, e.g. glucagon and vasoactive intestinal polypeptide (VIP). There is also an increased production of nitric oxide, which is a potent vasodilator.

## Answer 29

Antigen absorbed from the gut bypasses the liver in cirrhosis and also there is decreased function of the Kupffer cells in cirrhosis. Both of these allow antigen to stimulate the reticuloendothelial system in the spleen and lymph nodes to produce immunoglobulins.

## Answer 30

There is some evidence that fibrosis following liver damage is reversible. There are no drugs currently available to act on TIMPS.

*Further reading*
Benyon RC, Iredale JP (2000) Is liver fibrosis reversible? *Gut* **46**: 443–446.

## Answer 31

Nowadays the model for end-stage liver disease (MELD) is used as a predictor for liver transplantation in decompensated as well as compensated liver disease. It is based on serum creatinine, serum total protein and the international normalized ratio. The Child criteria are given in Table 7.1.

**Table 7.1** The Child criteria for end-stage liver disease

| | Child's grade | | |
| --- | --- | --- | --- |
| | A | B | C |
| Serum bilirubin (mg/dL) | <2 | 2–3 | >3 |
| Serum albumin (g/L) | 35 | 33 | <30 |
| Ascites | None | Easily manageable | Poorly controlled |
| Encephalopathy | None | None | Coma |
| 1-year survival | 85% | 30% | Approximately 5% |

## Answer 32

There is no treatment for cirrhosis *per se*. Antifibrotic drugs might be used in the future. At the present time:

1. Treat the cause, e.g. stop alcohol, remove iron in hereditary haemochromatosis.
2. Treat the complications:
   - portal hypertension and bleeding
   - ascites
   - portosystemic encephalopathy.
3. Refer for liver transplantation

## Answer 33

There is no role for liver dialysis in hepatic encephalopathy. We do not know the toxic products that cause encephalopathy but they are too small to be removed by dialysis.

## Answer 34

It is difficult to answer these questions because it depends on how abnormal the tests are when the patient stops drinking. Small elevations in liver enzymes, e.g. alanine transferase (ALT) 80 units, will take weeks, whereas an ALT of 200 units will take months. Indeed, the liver might be permanently damaged. The γ-GT rises in response to alcohol ingestion as well as liver disease. Moderate fat in the liver disappears within 3–4 months.

## Answer 35

Yes. Many patients with alcoholic liver disease also smoke, which is a risk factor for coronary artery disease.

## Answer 36

Decompensated liver disease is the term used to describe a patient with chronic liver disease (cirrhosis) who develops complications, e.g. bleeding, ascites or encephalopathy. In such a patient, the serum albumin is usually low and the patient might be jaundiced. The term 'liver cell failure' is sometimes used to describe acute hepatocellular failure or fulminant hepatic failure.

## Answer 37

Flapping tremors occur in hepatic encephalopathy and in chronic obstructive pulmonary disease with carbon dioxide retention. The mechanisms are unclear but ammonia seems to be involved in the tremor seen in hepatic encephalopathy.

## Answer 38

Yes; patients with hepatic encephalopathy can have basal ganglia signs without having Wilson's disease.

## Answer 39

In this age group, it is usual for the liver disease to present first. The liver disease is variable, from mild hepatitis to acute fulminant hepatitis and also cirrhosis. If there is any doubt, Wilson's disease should be further excluded by examination of the child and investigation of copper levels in the blood (low) or in the liver (high).

## Answer 40

No; the liver disease is variable. Wilson's disease should be excluded by appropriate investigations of copper metabolism.

## Answer 41

Oral contraceptives have been implicated as a cause of Budd–Chiari syndrome but, in general, drugs are not a cause of the pathology of this condition.

## Answer 42

A liver abscess can present as a very indolent condition and it can take a long time to diagnose. The best clues are a slight raised alkaline phosphatase and a raised serum vitamin $B_{12}$. You must have a high degree of suspicion.

## Answer 43

Hepatocellular carcinoma can be treated with surgical treatments:
- Resection
- Cryo-ablation
- Liver transplantation.

Non-surgical therapies are:
- Chemotherapy
- Radiation
- Chemoembolization
- Percutaneous ethanol injection
- Radiofrequency ablation.

Radiofrequency ablation involves passing a high-frequency alternating current to the tip of an electrode that is placed in the cancer lesion. The ions in the tissue follow the change in direction of the alternating current, producing frictional heat in the tissue to about 60°C. This produces a thermal energy lesion. It is useful for small tumours and can be carried out laparoscopically. In one series the patients' disease was controlled locally for 18 months (Barnett & Curley 2001).

*Reference*
Barnett CC, Curley SA (2001) Ablative techniques for hepatocellular carcinoma. *Seminars in Oncology* **28**: 487.

## Answer 44
Accidental rupture of a blood vessel will sometimes produce a small amount of blood, but usually there is no difficulty in differentiating from haemorrhagic ascitic fluid.

## Answer 45
No, this treatment is now never used.

## Answer 46
The problem with most antispasmodics is that they are not very effective *in vivo*. OK, you could try Buscopan, but don't be surprised if it doesn't work!

## Answer 47
This is a condition where there is increased tone in the sphincter measured by manometry. It is usually diagnosed after cholecystectomy when no stones can be found in the common bile duct to account for the persistent right upper quadrant pain. True Oddi dysfunction is rare and many patients have functional abdominal pain.

## Answer 48
In early pancreatitis, cathepsin B cleaves the trypsinogen activation peptide from trypsinogen within the acinar vacuoles, leading to activation of trypsin. Trypsin is normally inactivated quickly but in this case defence mechanisms are overwhelmed, leading to autodigestion of the pancreas. Experimentally, inhibition of cathepsin B reduces pancreatic damage.

## Answer 49
Octreotide has been used in the management of severe acute pancreatitis because there is a significant mortality associated with the condition and no very good treatment.

*Further reading*
Andriulli A et al. (1998) Meta-analysis of somatostatin, octreotide and gabexate mesilate in the therapy of acute pancreatitis. *Alimentary Pharmacology & Therapeutics* **12**: 257–245.

## Answer 50
In severe acute pancreatitis, pancreatic necrosis will release pancreatic enzymes into the peritoneal cavity; this causes paralytic ileus.

## Answer 51
Between 85 and 100% sensitive. A radioimmunoassay is available, which helps to overcome problems with the assay.

*Further reading*
Whitcomb DC (2006) Acute pancreatitis. *New England Journal of Medicine* **354**: 2142–2150.

## Answer 52
There is an association between smoking, chronic pancreatitis and PVD.

## Answer 53
No! There is no good explanation. It has been suggested that release of free fatty acids damages pancreatic acinar cells or capillary endothelium.

*Further reading*
Fortson MR et al. (1995) Clinical assessment of hyperlipidemic pancreatitis. *American Journal of Gastroenterology* **90**: 2134–2138.
Toskes PP (1990) Hyperlipidemic pancreatitis. *Gastroenterology Clinics of North America* **19**: 783–789.

## Answer 54
There is no consensus and further trials are being performed. If your patients cannot be included in a trial, there is some evidence for the use of 5-fluorouracil (5-FU) infusion after resection followed by gemcitabine.

## Answer 55
1. Beta-blockers are the best treatment but, if they cannot be used, endoscopic variceal banding is probably the best option.
2. Add in small doses slowly. Use spironolactone initially.

## Answer 56
It is said that hepatocellular carcinoma can occur without cirrhosis but it must be very rare.

## Answer 57
In chronic HBV infection, treatment is at present only given with abnormal transferases. Some patients with HCV infection are being treated with normal liver enzymes if liver histology is abnormal. Trials are still ongoing.

# Haematological disease 8

**Question 1**
What is favism?

**Question 2**
What is the haemoglobin content of reticulocytes and how can this be measured or determined?

**Question 3**
We are told that an erythrocyte sedimentation rate (ESR) above 100 mm/h has a limited differential diagnosis, mainly vasculitis, malignancy and granulomatous diseases. Could you explain whether that applies to an ESR after one hour or two?

**Question 4**
What causes a raised erythrocyte sedimentation rate (ESR)?

**Question 5**
What are the causes of very raised erythrocyte sedimentation rate (ESR)? I mean an ESR >100 mm/h. Is this test diagnostic in any disease besides polymyalgia rheumatica and giant cell arteritis?

**Question 6**
1. Does the erythrocyte sedimentation rate (ESR) rise with age?
2. Can an ESR of 50 mm/h in an 80-year-old female with no evidence of systemic disease be considered normal?

**Question 7**
1. What is a 'normal' erythrocyte sedimentation rate (ESR)? Is the equation of a normal ESR = age − 10, correct?
2. Would a normal ESR exclude a vasculitic cause in the case of stroke?

## Question 8
In which conditions is C-reactive protein (CRP) more informative than the erythrocyte sedimentation rate (ESR)?

## Question 9
What is the management of an isolated high ferritin (without any signs, symptoms or changes in the other blood investigations)?

## Question 10
Is the mean corpuscular volume (MCV) useful? What is the RDW and when is it used?

## Question 11
What is the significance of renal disease with respect to anaemia, if any?

## Question 12
Can anaemia be a differentiating point between muscle wasting and cachexia owing to another systemic disorder?

## Question 13
Anaemia of chronic disease does not respond to iron therapy, but there are trials studying the use of iron and erythropoietin (EPO). Could you tell me where to find more detailed information about these trials, and whether there have since been any further developments?

## Question 14
Is the deoxyuridine test helpful?

## Question 15
The Schilling test is very rarely performed. Why is this?

## Question 16
There is no extramedullary haematopoiesis in aplastic anaemia, why?

## Question 17
Why is the anaemia in aplastic anaemia, macrocytic?

## Question 18
Is vitamin $B_{12}$ absorbed passively from the jejunum?

## Question 19
What role does 'R' binder play in the absorption of vitamin $B_{12}$?

## Question 20
In pernicious anaemia, investigation of the serum shows an elevated level of gastrin. Why is it so?

## Question 21
1. Please explain the term Coombs' positive (direct and indirect) and negative haemolytic anaemia.
2. What are the principles of the Coombs' test?

## Question 22
How often is Aldomet (alpha methyldopa) associated with autoimmune haemolytic anaemia or hepatitis? Is a normal person, with a positive Coombs' test owing to previous treatment with this drug, safe to donate blood?

## Question 23
What is the mechanism of priapism in sickle-cell anaemia?

## Question 24
Is sickle-cell disease associated with any of the glomerular disorders?

## Question 25
What is the acute chest syndrome?

## Question 26
Patients with thalassaemia intermedia have recurrent leg ulcers and recurrent infections. What is the mechanism of this?

## Question 27
What is the mechanism of iron absorption from iron polymaltose complex and carbonyl iron?

## Question 28
Iron overload in patients with thalassaemia major should be checked by measuring the serum ferritin and hepatic iron stores. How are the hepatic iron stores measured? By liver biopsy? And does not the measurement of serum ferritin suffice?

## Question 29
In the investigation for paroxysmal nocturnal haemoglobinuria (PNH), are the sucrose haemolysis test and Ham's acid serum test commonly done? What are the principles behind these tests?

## Question 30
Why isn't the blood of polycythaemia vera patients, after repeated phlebotomies, used for transfusion purposes? Although it is a premalignant condition, the red cells do not contain a nucleus and thus transfusion of only pure red blood cells (RBCs) would be a great benefit.

## Question 31
What investigations are necessary to exclude secondary polycythaemia?

### Question 32
What is the management plan in a patient with secondary polycythaemia presenting with transient ischaemic attacks (TIA)?

### Question 33
Why do patients with polycythaemia vera have a tendency to bleed, even though 50% of them have an elevated platelet count?

### Question 34
In hyposplenic patients, what precautions are necessary for patients who intend to travel to Saudi Arabia for the Haj?

### Question 35
What is the mechanism of development of splenomegaly in chronic leukaemia?

### Question 36
In idiopathic thrombocytopenic purpura (ITP), thrombocytes are mainly destroyed in the spleen owing to an immune mechanism. Why, therefore, is there no splenic enlargement as there is with other diseases?

### Question 37
Where exactly is the Traub's space? How exact is the percussion of the Traub's space as a sign indicating the size of the spleen?

### Question 38
Can you please tell me the indications and complications of blood transfusion.

### Question 39
Several times I have read the phrase 'white blood cells elevated with a left shift'. I am wondering what 'left shift' or 'left deviation' stands for.

### Question 40
What is the clear definition of 'bleeding time' and 'clotting time'? And what are the applied differences between them?

### Question 41
What is the meaning of the international normalized ratio (INR) blood test?

### Question 42
What is the cause of moderate thrombocytopenia in Bernard–Soulier syndrome? It is a qualitative defect not a quantitative platelet disorder.

### Question 43
What is new about thrombopoietin?

## Question 44
What is the rationale behind the use of desmopressin in bleeding disorders?

## Question 45
What effect does the contraceptive pill have on the blood fibrinogen level and on blood coagulability?

## Question 46
Does standard (unfractionated) heparin in doses of 10 000–15 000 units/day need monitoring?

## Question 47
Is there an antidote for low-molecular-weight heparin (LMWH)? Can Enoxaprin be used?

## Question 48
1. What is the mechanism of the action of aprotinin?
2. What is the therapeutic window for aprotinin?
3. In a case of haemorrhagic stroke, how many days should aprotinin be prescribed for and what is the recommended dosage?

## Question 49
My question is, what are thrombophilia scan tests? Can we use these in patients on anticoagulant therapy?

## Question 50
In thromboembolic disorders, how is clopidogrel superior to aspirin?

## Question 51
What are the definitions for prothrombin time (PT) and partial thromboplastin time (PTT), and how are they different?

## Question 52
1. Why, in chronic disease anaemia, are serum iron and the total iron-binding capacity (TIBC) low?
2. Why, in sideroblastic anaemia with increased levels of serum iron, is the TIBC normal?

## Question 53
What is the red cell distribution width (RDW) value above which anisocytosis can be diagnosed?

## Question 54
Is anisocytosis diagnostic of iron deficiency anaemia?

## ANSWERS

### Answer 1
This is caused by the ingestion of fava beans. It can produce an acute haemolysis in patients with glucose-6-phosphate deficiency (G6PD). Others can enjoy the beans!

### Answer 2
The reticulocyte is a young erythrocyte without a nucleus. Over 90% of the reticulocyte's protein is haemoglobin. It is not normally measured.

### Answer 3
It applies to the ESR after 1 hour.

### Answer 4
A raised ESR is due to a rise in the large plasma proteins (e.g. fibrinogen or immunoglobulins). These proteins cause rouleaux formation when the cells clump together like a stack of coins and therefore fall more rapidly in a tube.

### Answer 5
A very high ESR occurs with myeloma and sometimes with malignancies where there is an increase in the plasma concentration of immunoglobulins. It can also occur in inflammatory conditions, e.g. rheumatoid arthritis and inflammatory bowel disease (IBD). It is never diagnostic but sometimes adds strong support to the clinical picture, e.g. polymyalgia, giant cell arteritis, rheumatic fever. Its main use is in monitoring the response to treatment, e.g. when using steroids for IBD, a fall in the ESR indicates a good response.

### Answer 6
1. There is a progressive rise with age. For example, in men aged 61–70 years the ESR is about 14; over 70, it is about 30. Women have slightly higher levels: aged 61–70 years the ESR is 20 and, over 70 it is 35.
2. An ESR of 50 mm/h is therefore abnormal in an 80-year-old but it is not usually worth pursuing beyond simple investigation (e.g. blood count). Do remember the various ways polymyalgia rheumatica can present, e.g. tiredness, loss of weight and often without the characteristic pain. It responds dramatically to steroids.

### Answer 7
1. Up to 20 mm in 1 hour. The equation is not helpful.
2. This makes it very unlikely but not impossible.

## Answer 8
CRP follows the clinical state of the patient much more closely in many inflammatory conditions, e.g. Crohn's disease. It is unaffected by anaemia. The CRP does not rise in systemic lupus erythematosus but the ESR does.

## Answer 9
Ferritin is an acute-phase protein and therefore will go up in inflammation, malignant disease or with acute liver necrosis. A high serum ferritin not associated with any of these should be investigated for possible hereditary haemochromatosis. Sending blood for genetic analysis of the *HFE* gene is now the best way to make this diagnosis.

## Answer 10
The MCV (normal range 80–96 fL) is useful in diagnosing the type of anaemia. A reading of <80 would suggest microcytic anaemia and >96 fL, macrocytic anaemia. The RDW (red blood cell distribution width) is the ratio of the width of the red cell over the MCV. It helps in the diagnosis of microcytosis but not macrocytosis. In a patient with anaemia, a raised RDW would favour iron deficiency and a normal RDW, thalassaemia.

## Answer 11
Anaemia is common in renal failure. The anaemia is often the normochromic, normocytic anaemia of chronic disease. The major cause of anaemia is a relative deficiency of erythropoietin. Other causes include bone marrow toxins, haemolysis, deficiency of haematinic factors *(K&C 6e, p. 667–668)*.

Recombinant human erythropoietin is effective treatment in these cases; remember to replenish iron stores to optimize therapy.

## Answer 12
Not really; anaemia can occur with cachexia associated with cancer and can also occur with muscle wasting associated with polymyositis.

## Answer 13
The statement is correct, the anaemia does not respond to iron therapy alone. EPO is used in anaemia of chronic disease, e.g. rheumatoid arthritis, chronic renal disease. The response can be dramatic so that iron must be made available, otherwise iron deficiency will occur.

*Further reading*
Remuzzi G, Inglefinger JR (2006) Correction of anemia – payoffs and problems. *New England Journal of Medicine* **355**; 2144–2146.

## Answer 14
The problem with this test is that it needs a bone marrow sample. It is useful, however, because it gives a rapid result for vitamin $B_{12}$ and folate

status, whereas the blood tests take more time. It is not used very often (*K&C 6e, p. 430*).

## Answer 15

Because radiolabelled vitamin $B_{12}$ is now unavailable in the UK.

## Answer 16

In aplastic anaemia there is damage to the stem cells, due to a number of causes including viruses and radiation. Damaged stem cells mean no haematopoiesis of any sort.

## Answer 17

In aplastic anaemia there are few red cells and the anaemia is usually normocytic. It can occasionally be macrocytic as the abnormal red cells can be big.

## Answer 18

Yes. Patients with pernicious anaemia who have no intrinsic factor can still be treated with vitamin $B_{12}$ orally by giving large amounts (2 mg per day), which are absorbed passively in the jejunum. There is a specific transport mechanism for vitamin $B_{12}$ in the ileum, which requires intrinsic factor as a cofactor.

## Answer 19

Vitamin $B_{12}$ is liberated from protein complexes in food by gastric enzymes and then bound to 'R' binder (a $B_{12}$ binding protein) from the saliva. This is similar to transcobalamin that is found in plasma. The bound $B_{12}$ is released by pancreatic enzymes and then becomes bound to intrinsic factor for absorption.

## Answer 20

In pernicious anaemia, there is atrophy of parietal cells and therefore no acid is produced. The gastrin level is raised as there is no negative feedback.

## Answer 21

1. In the direct Coombs' test, the patient's red cells are sensitized *in vivo*; the test is positive if agglutination occurs on the addition of antihuman globulin. In the indirect Coombs' test, normal red cells are sensitized *in vitro* by incubation with the patient's serum and again will be positive if there is agglutination on the addition of antihuman globulin.
2. The Coombs' test detects autoantibody on the surface of the patient's red cells.

## Answer 22

Twenty per cent of patients develop a positive Coombs' test with methyldopa but haemolytic anaemia is rare. Your normal person with previous drug treatment would not be able to donate blood because of problems with cross-matching and interference with agglutination tests. Hepatitis is rare.

## Answer 23

Veno-occlusion is the easy answer but the mechanism of priapism is not clearly understood in sickle-cell disease.

## Answer 24

Yes; focal glomerulosclerosis leads to end-stage renal disease.

## Answer 25

This describes the pulmonary complications that occur in sickle-cell disease. These include pneumonia, thrombosis causing infarctions in the chest or bone marrow and embolism due to fat. It occurs in about 30–50% of patients with sickle-cell disease and is the commonest acute problem in the chest.

## Answer 26

The mechanism is unclear but hypoxia due to anaemia has been suggested. Many are traumatic.

## Answer 27

These compounds will be broken down in the intestine. Ferrous iron is absorbed in the duodenum initially by attaching to a protein divalent metal transporter, which transports $Fe^{2+}$ into the cell where it is transported across the cell to reach the plasma or stored as ferritin (see reference). These compounds are, however, often passed intact beyond the point of iron absorption, the first part of the duodenum. Always prescribe simple iron preparations, e.g. ferrous sulphate.

*Further reading*
Fleming RE, Bacon BR (2005) Orchestration of Iron Homeostasis. *New England Journal of Medicine* **352**: 1741–1744.

## Answer 28

Iron stores have traditionally been assessed on liver biopsy – grams of iron per dry weight of liver. Magnetic resonance imaging is now the best technique. Measurement of serum ferritin will, however, suffice when monitoring treatment.

## Answer 29

Osmotic damage does not occur when normal red cells are exposed to isotonic sucrose. The low ionic strength of the solution enhances the binding of the complement components to the red cell membrane. PNH cells develop membrane defects and sucrose molecules enter the red cell, producing osmotic lysis; >5% lysis is positive. In the Ham test, PNH red cells are significantly lysed when exposed to acidified serum (>1% is positive). However, both these tests have now been replaced by flow cytometric analysis of red cells with anti-CD55 and anti-CD59 antibodies to the protein involved in the destruction of red cells by activated complement.

## Answer 30

Polycythaemia vera is a clonal cell disorder in which 5% of patients develop acute myeloid leukaemia. It is thus thought to be unwise to use this for blood transfusion. Red cells do not contain nuclei but even pure red cell concentrates still contain a few leukocytes that of course do contain nuclei.

*Further reading*
Campbell PJ, Green AR (2006) The Myeloproliferative disorders. *New England Journal of Medicine* **355**; 2452–2466.

## Answer 31

The secondary causes can sometimes be excluded with a history and examination. A renal ultrasound, an arterial $PO_2$ and carboxyhaemoglobin levels will exclude most causes of secondary polycythaemia.

## Answer 32

Treatment of the cause if possible; venesection may help. Aspirin 75 mg daily should be given.

## Answer 33

Platelets show a functional defect and haemorrhage causes death in 5% of patients.

## Answer 34

These patients should already have had pneumococcal and meningococcal group C vaccines. They should receive, in addition, the meningococcal polysaccharide vaccine (A, C, W, Y types).

*Further reading*
Gardner P (2006) Prevention of meningococcal disease. *New England Journal of Medicine* **355**: 1466–1473.

## Answer 35

The splenomegaly is due to a combination of extramedullary haemopoiesis and infiltration of the spleen with neutrophils.

## Answer 36

There is no explanation as to why the spleen remains the normal size. Presumably platelet destruction can occur without enlargement.

## Answer 37
The area of resonance overlying the gas bubble in the left lateral hemithorax. Its size and localization depend on the contents and position of the stomach. It is displaced downwards by an enlarged spleen. Compared with ultrasound scanning in one study, the sign was 62% sensitive and 72% specific.

## Answer 38
The main indication for blood transfusion is hypovolaemia due to loss of blood. The complications of blood transfusion are several (*K&C 6e, p. 460*) and include immunological causes (red cell and leucocyte incompatibility, anaphylactic reactions, graft versus host) and non-immunological (infection transmission, volume overload, thrombophlebitis). An avoidable cause is the transfusion of the wrong unit of blood.

## Answer 39
A blood film shows a shift to the left if there are relatively more young polymorphonuclear leucocytes present than normal. These young cells have more band forms within them, and in addition there are sometimes myelocytes present; for example this occurs in acute infection.

## Answer 40
The bleeding time measures platelet plug formation *in vivo*. Platelet function defects and low platelet numbers ($<80 \times 10^9$L) result in an increased bleeding time. Activated whole blood clotting time has been replaced by activated partial thromboplastin time (APTT), which is also known as the partial thromboplastin time with kaolin (PTTK) as a measure of clotting.

## Answer 41
The INR is the ratio of the patient's prothrombin time (PT) to a normal control when using the international reference preparation. PT tests are therefore standardized, whichever laboratory is used.

## Answer 42
The cause of the moderate thrombocytopenia in Bernard–Soulier syndrome is unclear. It is possibly related to ineffective or decreased thrombopoiesis.

## Answer 43
Thrombopoietin is a regulator of platelet function. Its clinical use is in cancer chemotherapy, both for solid tumours and for acute leukaemia, hopefully avoiding platelet transfusion. It is also being used in idiopathic autoimmune thrombocytopenia as second line therapy.

## Answer 44

Desmopressin is used in von Willebrand's disease to release von Willebrand factor from the endothelium. In platelet function disorders it might have an effect on platelet function. In haemophilia A, desmopressin produces a transient rise in factor VIII and is useful for treating bleeding episodes in mild haemophilia and as a prophylaxis before minor surgery.

## Answer 45

Factors V, VIII, X and fibrinogen levels are increased by ethinylestradiol, which can enhance thrombosis.

## Answer 46

Unfractionated heparin should always be monitored with activated partial thromboplastin time (APTT) to ensure adequacy of effect. The dose of 10 000–15 000 units will not be dangerous but might well be ineffective.

## Answer 47

Antidotes are not usually required for LMWH. Protamine (if used) is less effective than as an antidote against standard heparin. In patients at risk of bleeding, give LMWH twice daily instead of once. Enoxaprin is a LMWH.

## Answer 48

1. Aprotinin inhibits the activation of plasminogen to plasmin. It also inhibits kallikrein. These actions mean that aprotinin has an antifibrinolytic effect as well as inhibiting coagulation.
2. Aprotinin is given intravenously every hour in open heart surgery to reduce bleeding.
3. It is not recommended for haemorrhagic stroke.

## Answer 49

You cannot do thrombophilia scan tests on patients on anticoagulants.
   The thrombophilia tests are full blood count and coagulation screen, which will detect erythrocytosis, thrombocytosis and dysfibrinogenaemia and the possible presence of a lupus anticoagulant. Specific tests include; assay for antithrombin, protein C and S, molecular testing for factor V Leiden and for anticardiolipin antibodies.

## Answer 50

A number of studies have shown some slight benefit of clopidogrel over aspirin but with more bleeding, and it is more expensive. The question asks *how* is it superior? This is unclear, but is possibly due to a different site of action. Aspirin inhibits the enzyme cyclo-oxygenase (COX), resulting in reduced action of thromboxane $A_2$ ($TXA_2$). Clopidogrel affects the adenosine diphosphate (ADP) activation of the glycoprotein 11b/111a complex.

## Answer 51
The prothrombin time is prolonged with abnormalities of coagulation factors VII, X, V, II or I, liver disease or if the patient is on warfarin. The activated partial thromboplastin time (APTT) is prolonged with abnormalities of factors XII, XI, IX, X, V, II or I (not factor VII).

## Answer 52
1. The bone marrow contains iron but this is not released into the serum. The TIBC is low, as are levels of many circulating proteins. The mechanisms of these effects are unclear but are probably mediated by inflammatory cytokines.
2. In sideroblastic anaemia the TIBC might be high or normal, but not low.

## Answer 53
>15%.

## Answer 54
No; anisocytosis just means that the red cells are of different size on a blood film. This can occur with iron deficiency but also, for example, with thalassaemia.

# 9 Malignant disease

## QUESTIONS

**Question 1**
What is the meaning of 'opsoclonus' and does it always indicate malignancy?

**Question 2**
Does a greatly elevated lactate dehydrogenase (LDH) denote malignancy?

**Question 3**
Does a normal erythrocyte sedimentation rate (ESR) exclude malignancy in a patient complaining of feeling easily fatigued?

**Question 4**
Why is folic acid supplementation given just after the day of methotrexate administration? Can we give them simultaneously on the same day?

**Question 5**
Is hydroxyurea useful in the treatment of chronic myeloid leukaemia?

**Question 6**
What is the treatment of choice of mucosa-associated lymphoid tissue (MALT) lymphoma? Is the eradication of *Helicobacter pylori* enough? Does the positivity of CD2 rule out MALT lymphoma?

**Question 7**
Stage IIE Hodgkin's lymphoma is the 'involvement of one or more lymph node regions plus an extralymphatic site' and that stage IV is the 'involvement of one or more extralymphatic organs with or without

lymph node involvement'. What is the difference? Is 'site' different from 'organ' and, if so, what is 'site'?

## Question 8
1. What is Hodgkin's lymphoma?
2. What is the difference between Hodgkin's and non-Hodgkin's lymphoma?

## Question 9
Why is serum calcium elevated in patients suffering from lymphoma?

## Question 10
In a patient with suspected multiple myeloma, with pains in the back ribs, is the skull still the most sensitive site to observe bony lesions?

## Question 11
Please explain why the incidence of ovarian cancer (surface epithelial type)/carcinoma is low in women who take the oral contraceptive pill and who have undergone tubal ligation, compared with the general population?

## Question 12
What is the treatment of Kaposi's sarcoma?

## Question 13
How effective is a paracetamol and codeine phosphate combination in cancer pain therapy and ordinary pain therapy, and what is the difference in using them in cancer pain therapy?

## Question 14
What is meant by co-analgesic drugs in palliative care?

## Question 15
Is trastuzumab useful in all patients with metastatic breast cancer?

## Question 16
I have heard that Imatinib is useful in stromal cell tumours. Can you explain the mechanism?

## Question 17
Does monoclonal gammopathy of unknown significance (MGUS) progress to multiple myeloma?

## Question 18
Why do some cancers particularly metastase to bone?

## Question 19
What is the difference between lead time bias and length time bias.

## Question 20
Could lymphocytosis (lymphocytes: $4.4 \times 10^9$/L, representing 56% of total lymphocytic count) and not accompanied by any other haematological or systemic symptoms or signs except for mild weight loss (5–10% previous body weight) some 12 years ago, with no progression until now, be chronic lymphocytic leukaemia?

## ANSWERS

### Answer 1
Opsoclonus is characteristic of the paraneoplastic syndrome. It describes rapid, chaotic, conjugate, spontaneous eye movements that distort ocular fixation. It is associated with ataxia and other brain stem disturbances.

### Answer 2
It can do but a high LDH also occurs with haemolysis, liver disease and myocardial infarction.

### Answer 3
No; the ESR will usually be raised but this is by no means invariable.

### Answer 4
Folinic acid, not folic acid, is used to counteract the folate antagonist action of methotrexate and should be given 24 hours after the methotrexate and not at the same time.

### Answer 5
No.

### Answer 6
Low-grade gastric MALT lymphomas restricted to the mucosa or submucosa are often treated successfully by *H. pylori* eradication but others require surgery and chemotherapy. Try eradication therapy initially.

CD2 is associated with T and natural killer (NK) cells; MALT lymphomas are B cell lymphomas.

### Answer 7
'Site' and 'organ' mean the same most of the time. Sometimes, however, the site is clear (e.g. a mass in the epigastrium) without it being very obvious which organ is involved.

### Answer 8
Lymphomas are divided histologically into:
- Hodgkin's lymphoma: characteristically has Sternberg–Reed cells, together with a mixture of lymphocytes and histiocytes.
- Non-Hodgkin's lymphoma: does not have Sternberg–Reed cells but does have lymphoid tissue of various types depending on the type of lymphoma (*see K&C 6e, Table 9.18, p. 510*).

*Further reading*
Jaffe ES et al (eds) (2001) *WHO Classification of Tumours. Pathology and Genetics of Tumours of Haemopoietic and Lymphoid Tissues*. Lyon: IARC Press.

## Answer 9
Some lymphomas secrete 1,25-dihydroxycholecalciferol, which will raise the serum calcium level.

## Answer 10
No; an X-ray of the area of pain, e.g. the spine, would be the best test but a full skeletal survey, which would of course include the skull, is usually carried out in a patient suspected of having myeloma.

## Answer 11
The "Incessant ovulation theory" suggests that continuous ovulation in a nulliparous woman is associated with high frequency of malignant change. Ovulation is reduced by oral contraceptive treatment and is incomplete with tubal ligation, perhaps explaining the reduced frequency of ovarian cancer in these patients.

## Answer 12
Treatment of Kaposi's sarcoma depends very much on the site. Many do not need treatment but some need surgical treatment and others chemotherapy. This lesion is now much less common in patients with AIDS since the introduction of highly active antiretroviral therapy.

## Answer 13
Paracetamol and codeine phosphate as a combination at an adequate dosage is sometimes helpful in pain control. It is important that the drugs are given regularly. They can be useful in cancer pain when this is mild, making opiates unnecessary.

## Answer 14
These are drugs used in addition to opioids. Examples include NSAIDs, which are used with an opioid for bone pain, and anticonvulsant drugs, e.g. gabapentin, carbamazepine and pregabalin for neuropathic pain.

## Answer 15
No. It is only useful in patients who overexpress HER2 receptors. It is now being used in patients following surgery for early breast cancer, and in patients with metastatic disease. Trastuzumab is a member of the epidermal growth factor family.

## Answer 16
Stromal tumour cells have a mutation in the proto-oncogene, which leads to activation and cell surface expression of the tyrosine kinase KIT (CD117). Imatinib is a tyrosine kinase inhibitor and is also used in chronic myeloid leukaemia.

## Answer 17
Yes. Patients with a serum monoclonal protein concentration of
>1.5 g/dL that is IgA or IgM, and an abnormal serum free light chain
ratio (k: chains), are the most likely to develop multiple myeloma.

## Answer 18
Bone is a frequent site of metastasis due to its high blood flow. Tumour
cells also produce adhesins that bind them to marrow stromal cells. Bone
also contains growth factors, e.g. tumour growth factor beta (TGFβ).

## Answer 19
In 'lead' time bias, the diagnosis is made early, e.g. by screening so that
'survival time' appears longer. Death still occurs at the same time from
the genesis of the cancer.
    With 'length' time bias, a greater number of slowly growing tumours
are detected when screening asymptomatic individuals.

## Answer 20
Yes; chronic lymphocytic leukaemia can have a good prognosis (*see K&C
6e, Table 9.15, p. 507*). Lymphocytosis only has a median survival of
>10 years.

## QUESTIONS

### Question 1
How can gabapentin and carbamazepine act with a cervical disc prolapse?

### Question 2
Do patients with cervical spondylosis, experiencing neck pain and stiffness, benefit from putting on a neck collar? If so, for how long should the collar be worn?

### Question 3
What is indicated by a straightening of the lumbar spine with a loss of normal lordosis, and is there any relation to ankylosing spondylitis?

### Question 4
Can cervical spondylosis cause hypertonia in one upper limb?

### Question 5
Should a female patient, with mild congestive cardiac failure, microalbuminuria and cervical spondylosis receive IV vitamin D/analogues? Would this not increase the risk of calcium stones owing to the mild renal impairment? Would oral vitamin D be preferable?

### Question 6
What is the recommended treatment for spinal canal stenosis? Do carbamazepine or vasodilators have a role to play in its treatment?

### Question 7
What technique is used for injecting steroids locally in the case of carpal tunnel syndrome?

## Question 8

In a patient who has sustained an anterior cruciate ligament (ACL) knee injury and whose pain and swelling have subsided on conservative treatment, what are the chances of complications (e.g. osteoarthritis, fibrosis) from the torn ligament. Will the patient be able to lead a normal life?

## Question 9

Is either gapapentin or carbamazepine effective in the treatment of meralgia paraesthetica?

## Question 10

What is the clinical differentiation between Dupuytren's contracture and ulnar nerve palsy? Is it the absence of sensory deficit in the former? Are there any other differentiating factors?

## Question 11

1. Is a local corticosteroid injection in the palm effective in the case of Dupuytren's contracture?
2. Can Dupuytren's contracture occur in early or well-controlled diabetes, or is it more likely to occur in uncontrolled diabetes?

## Question 12

Besides cirrhosis of the liver and diabetes mellitus (DM), what other causes of Dupuytren's contracture are there? What is the pathophysiology behind it?

## Question 13

According to one of my lecturers, who is a very well-qualified doctor and orthopaedic specialist, there is an indirect connection between osteoarthritis and subclinical local infections (such as periodontal abscesses), changing the pH of bodily fluids. Can you explain this mechanism?

## Question 14

What do you mean by saying that in nodal osteoarthritis each joint is affected one at a time? Is it that each proximal interphalangeal (PIP) or distal interphalangeal (DIP) joint is affected alone, or that at any one time PIP or DIP joints are affected together in one or both hands?

## Question 15

What are the criteria for diagnosing osteoarthritis (OA) of the knee joint radiologically? Are changes to be expected with advancing age? To what extent would I consider it significant in those below 50 years of age? Would you give me some X-ray examples if possible?

## Question 16

1. In a young patient with osteoarthritis, does long-term treatment with paracetamol (acetaminophen) 500 mg/day, rather than ibuprofen 600 mg/day, lower the incidence of renal toxicity?
2. How great is the risk of renal toxicity with both these treatments?

## Question 17

In India, total knee replacements are being recommended for every case of severe osteoarthritis, without considering factors such as age, weight or medical condition. What are the correct indications for surgery?

## Question 18

Methotrexate therapy is usually begun in rheumatoid arthritis that doesn't respond to NSAIDs plus 40–120 mg methylprednisolone depot. If a remission is then induced, how long should methotrexate therapy be continued? Will the patient (now in remission) be given maintenance therapy?

## Question 19

What is the dose and regimen for folinic acid rescue after methotrexate in rheumatoid arthritis?

## Question 20

1. What are the indicators of remission in rheumatoid arthritis? Is it normalization of erythrocyte sedimentation rate (ESR) or clinical improvement?
2. Does the rheumatoid factor disappear during a remission of rheumatoid arthritis?

## Question 21

What is the relationship between rheumatoid arthritis and weight loss? Can treatment aid the weight loss at the same time as controlling the disease?

## Question 22

Can oral folic acid (1 mg/day) be used for high-dose methotrexate therapy with subsequent leucovorin rescue in the treatment of rheumatoid arthritis?

## Question 23

How often should a patient, on 8 mg/day methylprednisolone for the treatment of rheumatoid arthritis and on osteoporosis prophylaxis in the form of 1000 mg calcium and 400 IU vitamin D daily, have a dual energy X-ray absorptiometry (DXA) scan to detect the development of osteoporosis?

## Question 24

In what percentage of patients with psoriatic arthritis does the arthritis precede the onset of skin or scalp lesions?

## Question 25

1. Is reactive arthritis a synonym for Reiter's syndrome?
2. It is said that Reiter's disease has been related to *Chlamydia trachomatis* infection. Is this correct?

## Question 26

1. Is the response of an acutely inflamed joint to colchicine pathognomonic of gouty arthritis?
2. We are told that, other than clinical tests, joint fluid microscopy is the specific diagnostic test for gout. What does joint fluid microscopy reveal? Is it the same as a polarized light study revealing needle-shaped urate deposits?

## Question 27

In the prevention of gout, should allopurinol be used for life in a patient who is hypertensive, alcoholic and overweight?

## Question 28

Does a serum uric acid level of 5.7 mmol/L need treatment? Can it be significant with cholesterol levels of 213 mg/dL (5.5 mmol/L)? What is the treatment?

## Question 29

In the diet of patients suffering from gout, should tea, coffee or other compounds containing methylxanthine products be restricted?

## Question 30

1. When do joints that appear slightly swollen, but not warm, need to be tapped?
2. In what circumstances might an immunologically suppressed patient not mount a fever or not have heat around a septic joint?

## Question 31

What is the cause of Pott's disease?

## Question 32

One thing that often baffles me is that patients with systemic lupus erythematosus often suffer recurrent thrombosis due to lupus anticoagulants (antiphospholipid syndrome). How can an anticoagulant cause thrombosis?

## Question 33

Are elevated homocysteine levels an independent risk factor for progression of systemic lupus erythematosus (SLE)/scleroderma? Kindly suggest some references if possible.

## Question 34

1. What are the indicators of remission in systemic lupus erythematosus (SLE)? Is it the normalization of erythrocyte sedimentation rate (ESR) and the disappearance of antinuclear antibodies (ANA) and other antibodies, or is it clinical improvement?
2. During remission of SLE, do ANA and other antibodies disappear?

## Question 35

When should the use of cyclophosphamide in systemic lupus erythematosus (SLE) be commenced? What is the correct and safe dosage of cyclophosphamide?

## Question 36

1. Given the benefits of dexamethasone, which lacks any mineralocorticoid activity, why is this not prescribed in your book for diseases that require long-term steroid therapy, such as systemic lupus erythematosus or giant cell arteritis?
2. Does dexamethasone have more serious adverse effects than prednisolone? Why is it not generally preferred?

## Question 37

Would an elevated C-reactive protein (CRP) level, in association with a high erythrocyte sedimentation rate (ESR) and in the absence of infection and serositis, exclude the diagnosis of systemic lupus erythematosus?

## Question 38

How do steroids precipitate a crisis in patients with systemic sclerosis?

## Question 39

Are neck and face muscles commonly affected in poly- and dermatomyositis? Does this differ from the muscles that are affected with myasthenia gravis?

## Question 40

1. In dermatomyositis, what is the shawl sign?
2. How frequently is dermatomyositis associated with Gottron's papules?

## Question 41

How can cranial arteritis be diagnosed in the absence of any physical symptom or feature of the disease other than headache?

## Question 42
Do pulmonary manifestations in Behçet's syndrome present with pulmonary infiltrates in the upper zone of the lung?

## Question 43
1. Is Behçet's disease accompanied by an elevated erythrocyte sedimentation rate (ESR)? If so, how often?
2. Can Behçet's disease be diagnosed in a young adult with an ischaemic stroke and a history of almost weekly mouth ulcers that heal quickly, but with no other symptoms of Behçet's disease?

## Question 44
Mouth ulcers are too common to be a cardinal feature in the diagnosis of Behçet's disease. Are there any distinguishing features other than mouth ulcers that would confirm diagnosis?

## Question 45
Please explain how to diagnose familial Mediterranean fever. Is a diagnosis of exclusion still used or are there now more up-to-date tools for the diagnosis?

## Question 46
Is a leucocytoclastic reaction in a tissue biopsy specific for Henoch–Schönlein purpura or is it also associated with other problems?

## Question 47
What are the anatomical, histological and radiological differences between:
1. physis
2. metaphysis
3. epiphyseal disc
4. epiphyseal line?

## Question 48
Why does the serum alkaline phosphatase increase in bone disorders and in some other disorders?

## Question 49
What is the normal amount of calcium excreted in the urine in a 24-hour period?

## Question 50
Does hydrochlorothiazide have a prophylactic effect against osteoporosis?

## Question 51
How effective is parathyroid hormone in the management of osteoporosis? Please explain the mechanism.

## Question 52
1. What is the recommended treatment for severe osteogenesis imperfecta?
2. Where two siblings have already been born with severe osteogenesis imperfecta, what is the risk of subsequent children of the same parents being born with this condition?

## Question 53
Why does achondroplasia not affect the mandible (when all other bones are affected)?

## Question 54
If an elderly patient with rheumatoid arthritis who has been taking myocrisin (injectable gold) for several years presents with pancytopenia, should the gold treatment be stopped? If so, what treatment should replace it?

## Question 55
In a patient with dermatomyositis, what laboratory tests should be ordered to exclude systemic lupus erythematosus (SLE)?

## Question 56
What treatment is recommended for tarsal tunnel syndrome?

## Question 57
In a patient with documented antiphospholipid syndrome, should lupus anticoagulant be investigated for? If it is found to be present, will this necessitate the use of anticoagulants?

## Question 58
What are the findings to be looked for during routine fundus examination in patients on long-term chloroquine or any other antimalarial therapy for the treatment of systemic lupus erythematosus (SLE)?

## ANSWERS

### Answer 1
Both of these drugs are useful in neuropathic pain. Gabapentin has fewer side-effects and is becoming a first-line drug for nerve injury pain.

### Answer 2
A collar might be needed in the first 1–2 days. Fortunately, most patients are sensible enough not to wear them for any longer! They do not help in the long term.

### Answer 3
This does occur in ankylosing spondylitis. The lumbar spine can become straighter with the loss of the normal curvature (lordosis).

### Answer 4
Cervical spondylosis can lead to upper motor neurone signs. A spastic parapesis is the most common finding. There is often, in addition, evidence of a lateral disc protrusion with cervical root symptoms and signs.

### Answer 5
Yes. Oral vitamin D is always preferable, except sometimes in chronic renal failure. There seems, however, no reason for this particular patient to be given vitamin D at all.

### Answer 6
Spinal canal stenosis is diagnosed by the clinical history with confirmation of spinal cord compression on magnetic resonance imaging (MRI). The best treatment in these confirmed cases is surgery. Many patients with back pain are misdiagnosed because of slight but insignificant narrowing of the cord on MRI. Carbamazepine can be helpful in chronic back pain of undetermined cause. Vasodilators are of no help.

### Answer 7
This procedure should only be carried out by an experienced person who has been trained in the procedure. Nerve atrophy or necrosis can occur if steroids enter the median nerve directly.

The injection site is on the radial side of palmaris longus tendon; a mixture of lidocaine and steroid is used. The patient should be asked if he or she feels any distal sensation, which suggests that the needle is in the median nerve. Some operators use ultrasound to help to get the steroid into the tendon sheath.

## Answer 8

With good physiotherapy, patients can lead a normal life but in young athletes ACL repair is a better option. Osteoarthritis can occur in later life.

## Answer 9

Both drugs have been used with varying success. This self-limiting condition usually improves without medication.

## Answer 10

Dupuytren's causes flexion contracture of the fingers with thickening of the palmar fascia. Ulnar nerve palsy causes fixed flexion of the fingers, mainly the ring and little finger. Sensation can be lost.

## Answer 11

1. Triamcinolone is used in early and painful contractions with some benefit.
2. It occurs in 40% of diabetics; the incidence increases with age and duration of diabetes.

## Answer 12

It is also associated with alcohol abuse, DM, chronic obstructive pulmonary disease (COPD) and epilepsy. The pathophysiology is not understood.

## Answer 13

The pathogenesis of osteoarthritis is unclear and might well be different in different locations in the body. One explanation has been that it could be the result of occult infections. There is no good evidence to support this and most workers in this field think it unlikely.

*Further reading*
Poole AR, Howell DS (2001) Etiopathogenesis of OA. In: Moskowitz RW, Howell DS, Goldberg VM, Hankin HJ (eds) *Osteoarthritis: Diagnosis and Management*, 3rd edn. Philadelphia, Saunders, pp. 29–47.

## Answer 14

In osteoarthritis there is stuttering onset of inflammation affecting one joint at a time.

## Answer 15

Plain X-ray and skyline views of the patella are necessary. Joint space narrowing, osteophytes, subchondral radiolucencies and sclerosis are the classic signs of OA (Fig. 10.1). Osteophytes are the best predictor of knee pain. Some of these changes will be seen in a patient of advanced age and the significance must be correlated with the symptoms and signs. MRI is commonly used for more precise identification of the damage in osteoarthritis.

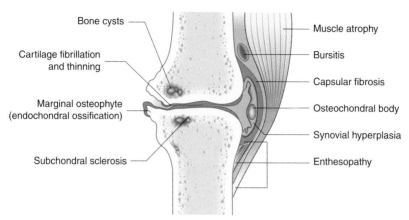

**Fig. 10.1** The early signs of osteoarthritis. Medial compartment narrowing results from cartilage thinning with subarticular sclerosis and marginal osteophyte formation.

## Answer 16
1. Acetaminophen is called paracetamol in many countries. It has no renal toxicity in therapeutic dosage. Ibuprofen is a non-steroidal anti-inflammatory drug (NSAID).
2. The prevalence of renal toxicity is relatively low but because of intensive usage, many persons are at risk.

## Answer 17
These are evolving and now many patients with stiff painful knees are being offered arthroplasty. There are, however, risks to these procedures and medical therapy should be provided first.

## Answer 18
Methotrexate therapy is often continued for many years (at least 10 years) if the patient remains well. Remember to check the liver biochemistry carefully and make sure that the prescription is for a once *weekly* dose.

## Answer 19
Give as calcium folinate 24 hours after the methotrexate, 15 mg orally every 6 hours for 2–8 doses.

## Answer 20
1. Both; clinical improvement is the most important but normalization of the ESR is also helpful.
2. Reduction in the rheumatoid factor titres occurs with disease-modifying anti-rheumatic drug (DMARD) therapy.

## Answer 21

'Active' rheumatoid arthritis makes people feel unwell so that they don't eat, and hence lose weight. Control of the disease will allow them to regain appetite. Be careful not to let the patient get overweight.

*Further reading*
Firestein GS (2006) Inhibiting inflammation in rheumatoid arthritis. *New England Journal of Medicine* **354**: 80–82.

## Answer 22

Methotrexate 7.5 mg weekly is used in rheumatoid arthritis. Folic acid 5 mg weekly can be given to reduce the side-effects. Calcium folinate (Leucovorin) is given after high-dose methotrexate to counteract the folate antagonist action of the drug.

## Answer 23

Yearly.

## Answer 24

Six per cent of patients have arthritis preceding the skin lesions.

## Answer 25

1. Reiter's describes a form of reactive arthritis where there is arthritis with urethritis, conjunctivitis, keratoderma blenorrhagica and circinate balanitis (*see K&C 6e, p. 568*).
2. Yes.

## Answer 26

1. Yes.
2. In this context, joint fluid microscopy refers to polarized light. In gout, crystals are needle shaped and negatively birefringent.

## Answer 27

In such a patient the hypertension should be treated. Drug therapy may well be needed but both reduction in weight and reduction in alcohol consumption are helpful in reducing blood pressure. Reduction in alcohol consumption (especially beer) will also reduce the number of attacks of gout.

The above measures are not always successful in preventing further attacks of gout, and in such a patient allopurinol will be required for life. However, a new drug, febuxostat, has become available.

*Further reading*
Becker MA et al. (2005) Febuxostat compared with allopurinol in patients with hyperuricaemia and gout. *New England Journal of Medicine* **353**: 2450–2461.

## Answer 28
Do not treat uric acid levels unless they are very high. You treat the symptoms produced by a raised uric acid; that is, gout. Cholesterol levels should be taken in isolation and not related to the uric acid level. The level of 213 mg/dL of cholesterol will require treatment in patients who have evidence of cardiovascular disease, usually with a statin.

## Answer 29
Yes, a diet that reduces total calories as well as cholesterol intake (avoiding offal, fish, shellfish, spinach and beer – all rich sources of purines) is advised. This can reduce the serum urate by 15%.

## Answer 30
Aspiration of a joint should always be undertaken if septic arthritis is a possibility (even if unlikely!). Aspiration is also useful in crystal arthritis. Constitutional symptoms are common but might not be present in severely debilitated patients and in patients on steroids or immunosuppressive agents.

## Answer 31
Tuberculosis of the spine.

## Answer 32
This paradoxical association between a prothrombotic state and the anticoagulant effect of antibodies is not fully understood.

*Further reading*
Lockshin MD, Erkan D (2003) Treatment of the antiphospholipid syndrome. *New England Journal of Medicine* **349**: 1177–1179.

## Answer 33
Yes; homocysteine levels are an independent risk factor for the progression of cardiovascular disease in SLE/scleroderma.

*Further reading*
Loscalzo J (2006) Homocysteine trials – clear outcomes for complex reasons. *New England Journal of Medicine* **354**: 1629–1632.
Svenungsson E et al. (2001) Risk factors for cardiovascular disease in systemic lupus erythematosus. *Circulation* **104**: 1887.

## Answer 34
High serum levels of ANA and anti-dsDNA with low complement do reflect disease activity. Clinical improvement is still the best indicator but a fall in antibody levels is helpful. They do not disappear. The ESR is raised in proportion to the disease activity.

## Answer 35

Many patients with SLE do well with little treatment. Cyclophosphamide is mainly used for lupus nephritis and vasculitis. For lupus nephritis, $0.75\,g/m^2$ has been used IV over 60 minutes.

## Answer 36

Dexamethasone is a highly potent glucocorticoid. Its main use is topically on the skin and by inhaler in asthma. Its high potency means that steroid side-effects occur very easily and dose can not be adjusted quickly; prednisolone is therefore usually preferred for chronic conditions.

## Answer 37

No. The ESR is raised; the CRP is usually normal but this is not reliable enough to be diagnostic.

## Answer 38

There is evidence to suggest that steroids precipitate a renal crisis in scleroderma. The mechanism is unclear but might be related to hypertension.

## Answer 39

Symmetric proximal muscle weakness is the most common presentation of polymyositis. Myasthenia gravis initially affects the eyes and other muscles controlled by cranial nerves. There can, however, be overlap.

## Answer 40

1. Involvement of the skin of the back of the neck, upper torso and shoulders in a shawl-like distribution.
2. 70–80% and is pathognomonic.

## Answer 41

Headache in an elderly person with a high erythrocyte sedimentation rate (ESR) is often all that is required. Without a rise in ESR the diagnosis is unlikely. Biopsy of the temporal artery is usually performed to confirm diagnosis; but remember, the inflammation is segmental and therefore might be negative.

## Answer 42

The findings are variable but nodular and reticular shadowing in the upper zone have been noted.

*Further reading*
Erkan F, Gul A, Tasali E (2001) Pulmonary manifestations of Behçet's disease. *Thorax* **56**: 572–578.

## Answer 43
1. Yes, in over 50% of cases. The C-reactive protein is also raised.
2. No; you need recurrent aphthous ulcers occurring more than three times per year, plus two of the following: genital ulcers, eye lesions, skin lesions, positive pathergy test.

## Answer 44
The international criteria for diagnosis of Behçet's state that the oral ulcers must recur more than three times per year. In addition to this, the ulcers are usually more extensive – genital ulcers, defined skin or eye lesions with a positive pathergy test (papule or pustular formation after a skin injury for e.g. by a needle) also occur.

## Answer 45
The diagnosis is still made on clinical grounds because identifying mutations in the *FMF* gene (*MEFV* on chromosome 16) is not always possible. The criteria used are:
- Intermittent episodes of fever.
- Serositis with abdominal pain and tenderness; pleuritis.
- The presence of amyloidosis.
- The therapeutic response to colchicine.
- Being of Mediterranean descent with sometimes a possible family history.

*Further reading*
Hatem El-Shanti et al (2006) Familial Mediterranean fever in Arabs. *Lancet* **367**: 1016–1024.

## Answer 46
A leucocytoclastic reaction also occurs in the condition known as leucocytoclastic vasculitis.

## Answer 47
- Physis: used for the growing part of a bone.
- Metaphysis: the site of advancing ossification adjacent to the epiphyseal cartilage.
- Diaphysis: shaft of bone.
- Epiphysis: extremity of bone with separate ossification centre. The 'line' is the junction of the epiphysis and diaphysis. The 'disc' is the band of cartilage between the epiphysis and diaphysis which is replaced by bone in later life.

## Answer 48
Osteoblasts are rich in alkaline phosphatase, so that in any bone condition with increased activity of osteoblasts, e.g. in the growing child

or in Paget's disease, there will be an increase in the serum alkaline phosphatase.

Alkaline phosphatase is also found in the placenta so that the serum level is raised in pregnancy.

## Answer 49

6.25 mmol (250 mg) in females to 7.5 mmol (300 mg) in men in 24 hours.

## Answer 50

Yes.

*Further reading*
Ray WA et al (1989) Long-term use of thiazide diuretics and risk of hip fracture. *Lancet* **1**: 687–690.

## Answer 51

Recombinant human parathyroid hormone peptide 1–34 (teriparatide) stimulates bone formation. It has been shown to reduce vertebral and non-vertebral fractures in postmenopausal women with established osteoporosis.

*Further reading*
Sambrook P, Cooper C (2006) Osteoporosis *Lancet* **367**: 2010–2018.

## Answer 52

1. Bisphosphonates are used for moderate and severe disease (see reference).
2. The risk is 1:2 but may be less with decreased penetrance.

*Further reading*
Rauch F, Glorieux FH (2004) Osteogenesis imperfecta. *Lancet* **363**: 1427.

## Answer 53

This is not known.

## Answer 54

The gold treatment should be stopped. If there is 'active' disease then referral to a rheumatologist for possible consideration of infliximab is recommended.

## Answer 55

The differentiation is usually not a problem. The proximal muscle weakness is unusual in SLE. The creatine kinase is usually raised in dermatomyositis. Double-stranded DNA is specific for SLE but is present in only 50% of cases. Remember the overlap syndrome (*see K&C, 6e, p. 581*) in which features of both diseases can be present.

## Answer 56
Arch supports and wider shoes often help, and NSAIDs are useful for pain and inflammation. Steroid injection into the tendon is also effective; surgery is the last resort.

## Answer 57
The lupus anticoagulant is usually looked for but treatment of the syndrome does not depend entirely on this. Treatment is given if the patient has had a thrombotic episode or, occasionally, if there are high levels of antibody and lupus anticoagulant present.

## Answer 58
All patients should have near visual acuity of each eye performed before treatment and annually on treatment. Patients who have any visual symptoms should be seen immediately. Fundoscopy will show round, pigmented lesions near the macula but it is the visual acuity and visual field examination that will give the first clue.

# 11 Renal disease

## Question 1
How do you calculate the plasma creatinine clearance value at the bedside, by body weight?

## Question 2
Can you tell me whether administering low doses of dopamine to increase renal blood flow is today considered obsolete?

## Question 3
Why does haemoglobinuria cause anuria?

## Question 4
I am confused over the use of a 'high-protein diet' in the management of nephrotic syndrome. You say it confers no advantage, but the *Oxford Handbook of Clinical Medicine* advocates its use and Davidson's *Principles and Practice of Medicine* says it is even dangerous as it could lead to renal damage. Which one should I choose, assuming I see the question in an MCQ?

## Question 5
Is albumin infusion contraindicated in nephrotic syndrome? If not, then what are the indications?

## Question 6
Listed under the drug causes of nephrotic syndrome, it has been stated that high doses of captopril can induce an immune-complex-mediated membranous glomerulonephritis. If a patient with nephrotic syndrome has hypertension, is it detrimental to give captopril as a treatment for his hypertension? Could this exacerbate the patient's nephrotic syndrome?

## Question 7
Please explain the pathophysiology of ascites in the nephrotic syndrome?

## Question 8
Does the nephritic syndrome cause hyperkalaemia? I don't seem to be able to find a definitive answer in the textbooks that I have consulted.

## Question 9
You say that the investigation of first choice for urinary tract infections (UTIs) in males or children, or recurrent UTIs in females, is intravenous urography (IVU); in *Oxford Handbook of Clinical Medicine* it is ultrasound (US). Which is best?

## Question 10
1. Other than amoxicillin, what other orally administered drug is recommended for the treatment of a urinary tract infection (UTI) caused by enterococcus?
2. What is the recommended dosage for antibiotics in the prophylactic treatment of recurrent UTI in pregnancy? Is amoxicillin + clavulanic acid safe to use during pregnancy?

## Question 11
What is the advantage of intermittent self-catheterization over an indwelling catheter? How is bladder training done while on an indwelling catheter?

## Question 12
Kindly tell me about the role of pulse wave velocity (PWV) in early diagnosis of arteriosclerosis. How is it useful in cardiac, diabetic and renal medicine?

## Question 13
You say that no convincing evidence was found that chronic hyperuricaemia causes nephropathy and nor can it be corrected by allopurinol. However, some patients we see have high serum uric acid and creatinine, which both come down with allopurinol. Please comment.

## Question 14
Can aspirin cause analgesic nephropathy? If yes, then how could we justify its use in primary prevention of coronary artery disease (CAD), even in high-risk patients? I have read that regular use of analgesics for 3 years could cause analgesic nephropathy.

## Question 15
What is the probability that a patient on a moderate daily dose of non-steroidal anti-inflammatory drugs (NSAIDs; ibuprofen 800 mg once daily for tension headache) will develop analgesic nephropathy?

## Question 16
Do daily doses of paracetamol with the dosage range of 1 g/day cause analgesic nephropathy. If so, after what length of time?

## Question 17
Allopurinol is used for the treatment of uric acid stones; it is also one of the aetiologies of renal calculi. Could you please explain its actual effect.

## Question 18
Why should we avoid angiotensin-converting enzyme (ACE) inhibitors as hypertensive therapy in the presence of renal artery stenoses? How can they lead to acute renal failure? What else can we prescribe for this patient to regulate the hypertension?

## Question 19
Is the use of angiotensin-converting enzyme (ACE) inhibitors contraindicated in cases of unilateral renal artery stenosis?

## Question 20
1. How effective is renal duplex in detecting renal artery stenosis?
2. Is magnetic resonance angiography superior to renal duplex in detecting renal artery stenosis?

## Question 21
How accurate is ultrasonography in detecting renal calculi?

## Question 22
Please explain the most effective way to manage a case of intrauterine fetal unilateral hydronephrosis in the 32nd week of pregnancy.

## Question 23
In renal failure, why does oedema first occur in the periorbital area and nowhere else?

## Question 24
How does sodium valproate decrease serum urea concentration and GI bleed increases it?

## Question 25
1. What clinical information can be obtained by checking the blood urea nitrogen (BUN) level that cannot be obtained by checking the blood urea and serum creatinine alone?
2. What is the signifying difference between blood urea and BUN?

## Question 26
1. Does uraemia cause dysentery with blood and mucus mixed with the stools?
2. Is it correct to use the term 'uraemic dysentery'?
3. Does uraemia cause finger clubbing?

## Question 27
What are the causes of a low serum creatinine?

## Question 28
Why does oliguria occur in the early stages of acute tubular necrosis (ATN)?

## Question 29
Is renal impairment induced by lithium therapy in bipolar affective disorders irreversible? How often does it occur?

## Question 30
Can you please explain why a patient with chronic renal failure (CRF) might present with either oliguria or polyuria?

## Question 31
What are uraemic frost conditions?

## Question 32
What is the role of terlipressin or novapressin in the management of hepatorenal syndrome?

## Question 33
What is the rationale of angiotensin-converting enzyme (ACE) inhibitors in chronic renal disease?

## Question 34
What procedure is recommended for post renal transplant if this is the second graft?

## Question 35
Do the cysts in autosomal-dominant polycystic kidney disease (PCKD) undergo malignant transformation and in what percentage?

## Question 36
In a 69-year-old patient with a 2-cm hard prostatic nodule on digital rectal examination, what is the more appropriate way to make a definitive diagnosis of prostate cancer: prostate biopsy or serum prostate-specific antigen (PSA)?

## Question 37
A 50-year-old patient complains from slight lower urological symptoms (mild difficulty in urination). By digital rectal examination a mass of (+1) hypertrophy can be palpated. His family history contains cases of prostate cancer (in some relatives). What is the next investigation to do in this patient?
- Titration of serum prostate-specific antigen (PSA): Is it useful in such a patient? Why?
- Transrectal ultrasound (TRUS)?
- TRUS-guided needle biopsy?

## Question 38
What are the causes of urinary incontinence in the elderly?

## Question 39
For how long could urinary retention persist after major gastrointestinal tract surgery? Will cholinesterase inhibitors be of benefit in enhancing emptying of the bladder?

## Question 40
1. What are the possible causes of a large, white kidney?
2. What is the physiological significance of a giant cell?

## Question 41
What is the amount of 24-hour urinary albumin excretion above which a diabetic patient is said to have microalbuminuria?

## Question 42
How is forced diuresis induced in cases of prerenal failure?

# ANSWERS

## Answer 1
The Cockcroft–Gault method is widely used:

$$\text{Creatinine clearance} = (140 - \text{age}) \times \text{bodyweight (kg)} \times 1.23 \text{ (males) or}$$
$$1.04 \text{ (females)}/\text{serum creatinine } (\mu\text{mol}/\text{L})$$

Nowadays, the glomerular filtration rate (GFR) is calculated automatically on read-outs from laboratory machines. The Modification of Diet in Renal Disease (MDRD) is another measure that uses serum creatinine level, sex and ethnicity to calculate estimated glomerular filtration rate (eGFR). A further formula is the National Kidney Foundation clinical practice guidelines formula.

*Further reading*
Stevens LA et al. (2006) Assessing kidney function – measured and estimated glomerular filtration rate. *New England Journal of Medicine* **354**: 2473–2483.

## Answer 2
The effect of low-dose dopamine on renal blood flow has been questioned. The effect of increasing urine output is now thought to be largely due to the rise in cardiac output. Low-dose dopamine is still used and is not obsolete, as it often helps in shock whatever the mechanism.

## Answer 3
Haem pigment casts obstruct the tubules.

## Answer 4
A high-protein diet confers no advantage and should not be used. Always choose Kumar and Clark!

## Answer 5
No, albumin infusion is not contraindicated but its effect is transient. It is sometimes used in diuretic-resistant nephrotic syndrome patients with an albumin of less than 20 g/L. It is combined with diuretic therapy, e.g. furosemide. There is no good evidence, however, of its clinical usefulness.

## Answer 6
Proteinuria sufficient to cause the nephrotic syndrome has been described with captopril. Angiotensin II receptor antagonists would be better in the circumstances you describe.

*Further reading*
Tryggvason K et al. (2006) Hereditary proteinuria syndromes and mechanisms of proteinuria. *New England Journal of Medicine* **354**: 1387–1401.

## Answer 7

Expansion of the interstitial compartments (i.e. the peritoneal cavity in ascites) is secondary to the accumulation of sodium in the extracellular compartment. Sodium retention occurs because of increased $Na^+/K^+$-ATPase expression and activity in the cortical collecting duct. Additional factors include elevated tumour necrosis factor alpha (TNF-$\alpha$) levels and an increase in circulating atrial natriuretic protein (ANP) levels, which change capillary permeability.

## Answer 8

Acute nephritic syndrome with acute renal failure causes hyperkalaemia. Nephrotic syndrome does not, unless acute renal failure supersedes.

## Answer 9

IVU shows the anatomical detail better than US and was regarded by many as first choice. US does not show pelvicalyceal anatomy as well but it does rule out major abnormalities, e.g. obstruction, and many urologists do not now use IVU. US followed by contrast-enhanced computed tomography has become more common.

## Answer 10

1. Trimethoprim, an oral cephalosporin, or ciprofloxacin is used. A pretreatment urine culture should be obtained if possible and the treatment can then be changed according to bacterial sensitivities and clinical response.
2. Dose: amoxicillin 250 mg every 8 hours for 5 days. Co-amoxiclav is safe in pregnancy. Bacteruria should always be treated in pregnancy and shown to be eradicated.

## Answer 11

This depends on the clinical need. Intermittent catheterization is associated with fewer urinary infections. Bladder training involves closing off the catheter intermittently for increasing lengths of time.

## Answer 12

Pulse-wave velocity is an indicator of arterial stiffness measured by Doppler ultrasound. Its use is not widespread but some studies suggest that it indicates atherosclerosis independent of blood pressure and might therefore be of prognostic value. The properties of the arterial wall, its thickness and the arterial lumen diameter are factors that influence PWV.

## Answer 13

There is evidence to suggest that chronic hyperuricaemia causes nephropathy, but this does not happen as often as was originally thought.

## Answer 14
Aspirin in large doses used over a long time can produce analgesic nephropathy; this was well described in Australia some years ago. In small doses, e.g. 75–150 mg a day, aspirin appears very safe and should be used for primary prevention in high-risk patients.

## Answer 15
Renal lesions are rare and at this dose and frequency the patient is very unlikely to develop analgesic nephropathy.

## Answer 16
No.

## Answer 17
Allopurinol blocks the enzyme xanthine oxidase which converts xanthine into urate. The level of urate in the blood falls, as does the amount in the urine. It does not cause uric acid stones.

## Answer 18
In renal artery stenosis there is reduced renal perfusion, reduced transglomerular pressure and reduced glomerular filtration rate (GFR), which leads to acute renal failure. The response is intrarenal activation of the renin–angiotensin system, which leads to efferent arterial vasoconstriction. This restores transglomerular pressure and glomerular filtration rate. Angiotensin-converting enzyme (ACE) inhibition or blockade prevents angiotensin release and stops the resultant response. Use other drugs, such as nifedipine or a beta-blocker.

## Answer 19
Yes.

## Answer 20
1. Duplex scanning compared to arteriography is over 90% sensitive and specific.
2. Yes, and this is now best practice for the diagnosis.

## Answer 21
Small calculi might be missed.

## Answer 22
This is a very specialized area and consultation with a paediatric urologist is essential. In general, hydronephrosis is being detected more frequently as routine ultrasonography becomes more common. In most cases, fetal surgery has not been beneficial. The most common cause of hydronephrosis is pelviureteric obstruction, which does not generally

impair renal function. Expectant management with follow-up at 2-monthly intervals is the best approach.

## Answer 23

In renal failure, oedema is due (as in other conditions) to fluid retention. The oedema is generalized but is often first noticed in the lax tissues around the eyes (periorbital area).

## Answer 24

Blood is protein and therefore contains nitrogen, which is converted to urea; hence the rise in urea concentration with a gastrointestinal bleed. It is unclear whether sodium valproate does decrease the urea concentration but it does have a number of metabolic effects. Valproate produces anorexia, which reduces protein intake, and this could lower the serum urea. Of course, you also get a low urea in severe liver disease, which very rarely occurs with sodium valproate. Sodium valproate also raises the ammonia level, again rarely, which could affect the urea level.

## Answer 25

BUN is shorthand for blood urea nitrogen; that is the blood urea. We now do not measure blood urea, we measure serum or plasma urea. There is, therefore, no difference between the BUN and the serum urea.

## Answer 26

1. No.
2. No.
3. No.

## Answer 27

Small body mass.

## Answer 28

There are many mechanisms but vasopressin levels are elevated so that free water and urea excretion are reduced. Angiotensin II and aldosterone are also increased, reducing sodium and hence water excretion.

## Answer 29

Renal impairment is usually reversible but cases have been reported in which progression occurs when lithium has not been stopped immediately. It is uncommon if lithium therapy is monitored with serum levels.

## Answer 30

CRF can present with polyuria, which is due to failure of tubular reabsorption. When depression of glomerular filtration occurs, oliguria tends to replace polyuria. Because tubular dysfunction always accompanies glomerular disease to some extent, the urine output is not a useful guide to renal function. The oedema occurs because of increased sodium tubular reabsorption.

## Answer 31
This is a term used for the appearance of the skin, literally 'a frost', which occurs only in terminal renal failure. In the age of dialysis and renal transplantation it is now not seen in developed countries.

## Answer 32
Terlipressin has been most used and a response occurs in about 60% of patients, usually over a few days. It improves circulatory function by vasoconstriction of the dilated splanchnic arteries, which subsequently suppresses the activity of the endogenous vasoconstrictor systems, resulting in increased renal perfusion. The response, however, is frequently transient: most patients with the hepatorenal syndrome require liver transplantation.

## Answer 33
ACE inhibitors reduce intraglomerular pressure and proteinuria as well as blood pressure in chronic renal failure. They slow progression of the renal disease (Box 11.1).

---

**Box 11.1 Renoprotection**

**Goals of treatment**
- Blood pressure < 120/80 mmHg
- Proteinuria < 0.3 g/24 hours

**Treatment**
**Patients with chronic renal failure and proteinura >1 g/24 hours**
- Angiotensin-converting enzyme inhibitor increasing to maximum dose
- Add angiotensin receptor antagonist if goals are not achieved*
- Add diuretic to prevent hyperkalaemia and help to control blood pressure
- Add calcium-channel blocker (verapamil or diltiazem) if goals not achieved

**Additional measures**
- Statins to lower cholesterol to < 4.5 mmol/L
- Stop smoking (threefold higher rate of deterioration in chronic renal failure)
- Treat diabetes (HbA$_{1C}$ < 7%)
- Normal protein diet (0.8–1 g/kg bodyweight)

---

* In type 2 diabetes, start with an angiotensin-receptor antagonist

*Further reading*
Herbert LE (2006) Optimising ACE-inhibitor therapy for chronic kidney disease. *New England Journal of Medicine* **354**: 189–191.

## Answer 34

If by 'procedure' you mean immunosuppressive regime, then for a high-risk patient (e.g. after a previous graft), CD25 monoclonal antibodies (e.g. basiliximab or dacluzimab) are used as induction therapy, followed by mycophenolate (replacing azathioprine) and tacrolimus.

## Answer 35

Malignant transformation does not occur in PCKD.

*Further reading*
Perrone R (2006) Imaging progression in polycystic kidney disease. *New England Journal of Medicine* **354**: 2181–2183.

## Answer 36

Prostate biopsy. A histological diagnosis is essential; the Gleason Scoring System, which guides treatment and includes prognosis, depends on this.

## Answer 37

The risk of prostate cancer is approximately two-fold in men with first-degree relatives affected. There is perhaps a trend to an increase when other relatives are affected. In the particular instance of the 50-year-old man the correct procedure is rectal ultrasound-guided needle biopsy. The serum prostate-specific antigen (PSA) is useful in that:
- a PSA < 4 is normal
- a PSA 4.1–10 means the cancer is confined to the prostate
- a PSA > 10 indicates the likelihood of extraprostatic extension by up to 30- to 40-fold.

## Answer 38

The causes of urinary incontinence are represented by the acronym DIAPPERS:
- **D**elirium
- **I**nfection
- **A**trophic urethritis
- **P**harmacological (drugs)
- **P**sychological
- **E**xcess urine output (e.g. diabetes, congestive cardiac failure)
- **R**estricted mobility
- **S**tool impaction

*Further reading*
Resnick NM (1996) Geriatric incontinence. *Urological Clinics of North America* **23**: 55.

## Answer 39
Urinary retention can persist for days, particularly in elderly men with enlarged prostate glands. After 24 hours, catheterization is usually performed. Cholinesterase inhibitors are now not used because of side-effects.

## Answer 40
1. Amyloid involvement of the kidneys produces enlarged, pale kidneys.
2. Giant cells are due to the fusion of activated macrophages and are seen in chronic inflammation, e.g. tuberculosis.

## Answer 41
Normal people excrete 30 mg of albumin in 24 hours. Excretion of 30–300 mg is called microalbuminuria. Above 300 mg in 24 hours can be detected by dipstix and is termed 'albuminuria'.

## Answer 42
Prerenal failure is due to hypovolaemia, hypotension or fluid and electrolyte depletion. You need, therefore, to replace fluids initially with 0.9% saline with potassium (20 mmol). Monitor the pulse, blood pressure and venous pressure. A diuresis will occur when volume repletion has taken place.

# 12 Water, electrolytes and acid–base balance

## QUESTIONS

### Question 1
1. Why do conditions that cause retention of sodium, such as cardiac failure, result in low serum sodium?
2. What is meant by 'free water'?

### Question 2
Why is there a difference in the pattern of oedema in nephrotic syndrome and cardiac oedema? How is it related to the interstitial spaces and all that? I am confused.

### Question 3
Why is there a difference in the clinical presentation of oedema due to renal failure and oedema due to cardiac failure, and how is this related to the loose nature of the interstitial tissue in the periorbital area? The answer given was that it is because, in cardiac failure, there is orthopnoea and the most dependent portion in this case is the legs, which is why the oedema occurs there. You also mentioned that in renal failure there is no orthopnoea and the patient doesn't have to sit up, hence the difference. This does not seem to take into account right ventricular heart failure (RVF), where there is no question of orthopnoea. Pedal oedema is found in right ventricular failure. Is the answer not that, in congestive heart failure (CHF) there is pump failure (and the heart cannot pump blood against gravity) hence oedema in the dependent areas, whereas in renal failure there is no pump failure and the heart does not lose its capacity to pump blood against gravity. The oedema in this case develops in those tissues that have a loose interstitium, one such site being the periorbital area of the face. This is the reason for the difference in clinical presentation.

### Question 4
What treatment is recommended for recurrent attacks of generalized swelling, with angio-oedema, in a middle-aged female patient?

## Question 5

Is an osmotic diuresis, due to hyperglycaemia for instance, a cause of both hyponatraemia and hypernatraemia. Please explain how this can be the case.

## Question 6

What is the mechanism of $\beta_2$-agonists (albuterol) in correcting hyperkalaemia in emergency? How does it cause a shift of potassium?

## Question 7

Why do we give sodium lactate along with sodium bicarbonate in acidotic patients? How does sodium lactate then act?

## Question 8

How does hypochloraemia alone cause a metabolic alkalosis?

## Question 9

I have read the part concerning acid–base imbalances and I would like to ask about two things:

1. Why is there a higher concentration of anions (18) on measuring the anion gap while there is a high concentration of immeasurable anions? I would have expected a higher concentration of cations because most of them are measurable.
2. Could you explain to me in more details how $NaCO_3$ loss or HCl retention could lead to normal anion gap acidosis?

## Question 10

What is the exact formula for calculating the serum anion gap?

## Question 11

What is the role of IV saline in the management of a cirrhotic patient with a serum sodium of 120 mmol/L?

## Question 12

Why do we give calcium gluconate to a patient with severe hyperkalaemia?

## Question 13

Can you explain the respiratory alkalosis and metabolic acidosis in salicylate poisoning?

## Question 14

In an elderly patient with oedema due to heart failure, which is the best diuretic to start treatment with? Some books recommend thiazides whereas others use loop diuretics.

## ANSWERS

### Answer 1

1. One explanation is the non-osmotic release of antidiuretic hormone (ADH), due to arterial underfilling causing the retention of water and a dilutional hyponatraemia. A second explanation is that reduced delivery of chloride to the diluting segment of the ascending loop of Henle because of avid reabsorption of sodium and chloride in the proximal tubule. This results in a reduced ability to generate 'free water' and produce a dilute urine so hyponatraemia occurs due to water excess.
2. The term 'free water' is a concept that is used to describe the movement of water independent of sodium.

### Answer 2

In all conditions associated with oedema there is increased extracellular volume associated with renal sodium chloride retention.

The oedema in all conditions is usually in the ankles in all patients but this depends on body position. Patients with the nephrotic syndrome are not usually breathless and so lie flat and the oedema occurs in the face. The reverse is true for cardiac failure.

### Answer 3

We are obviously going to disagree. Can we give you an example? In nephrotic syndrome, patients have periorbital oedema in the morning because of lying flat; in heart failure, the patient cannot lie flat because of orthopnoea. As oedema progresses, all spaces are eventually filled with fluid.

### Answer 4

This sounds like idiopathic oedema of women. It might respond to diuretics. Antidiuretic hormone (ADH) acts on vasopressin ($V_2$) receptors located on principal cells. ADH promotes water reabsorption in the collecting ducts and this might be a factor in the cause of the oedema. $V_2$ receptor antagonists should soon become available.

*Further reading*
Hays RM (2006) Vasopressin antagonists – progress and promise. *New England Journal of Medicine* **355**: 2146–2148.

### Answer 5

Hypernatraemia is due to loss of $Na^+$ and water with the osmotic diuresis. This causes dehydration and hypernatraemia. Hyponatraemia occurs because antidiuretic hormone (ADH) stimulates thirst; excess water compared to sodium is drunk, and hyponatraemia occurs.

## Answer 6

$\beta_2$-adrenergic receptors increase the activity of the sodium–potassium ATPase pump in the cell membrane. This is followed by the excretion of excess potassium in the urine.

## Answer 7

Sodium lactate intravenous infusion is obsolete for the treatment of metabolic acidosis. It carries the risk of lactic acidosis and should not be used.

## Answer 8

If chloride is lost either through the kidney or via the stomach, there is a preferential absorption of bicarbonate in the distal tubule. This leads to metabolic alkalosis.

## Answer 9

1. Normally there is an anion gap of approximately 12 mmol/L. Albumin normally makes up the largest portion of these unmeasured anions.
2. The loss of bicarbonate, e.g. from the gastrointestinal tract, is initially compensated but eventually the increased loss of bicarbonate leads to hydrogen ion excess; that is, acidosis (Fig. 12.1).

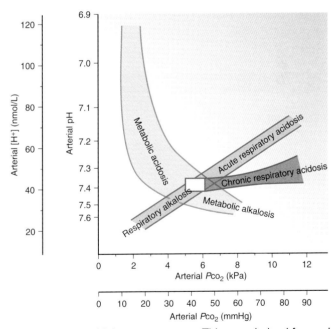

Fig. 12.1 The Flenley acid–base nomogram. This was derived from a large number of observations in patients with 'pure' respiratory or metabolic disturbances. The bands show the 95% confidence limits representing the individual varieties of acid–base disturbance. The central white box shows the approximate limits of arterial pH and $P_{CO_2}$ in normal individuals.

## Answer 10

Anion gap is calculated using serum concentrations as:

$$(Na^+ + K^+) - (Cl^- + HCO_3^-)$$

The normal value is 6–12 mmol/L.

## Answer 11

The initial management is with water restriction as the hyponatraemia is dilutional. IV saline therapy depends on:
- the rapidity of the development of hyponatraemia
- whether the patient is symptomatic.

In most patients with liver disease, the onset is slow and the patient is consequently asymptomatic; Hypertonic saline 3% should only be given to patients with neurological symptoms and signs and must be given extremely slowly so that the change in serum sodium should not exceed 15 mmol over 48 hours.

## Answer 12

Calcium ions protect the cell membrane from the effects of hyperkalaemia although they don't alter the potassium concentration. The correction of this acute hyperkalaemia is shown in Box 12.1.

---

**Box 12.1 Correction of severe hyperkalaemia**

**1. Immediate**
**Attach ECG monitor and IV access**
**Protect myocardium**
- 10 mL of 10% calcium gluconate IV over 5 min
- Effect is temporary but dose can be repeated after 15 min

**Drive $K^+$ into cells**
- Insulin 10 units + 50 mL of 50% glucose IV over 10–15 min followed by regular checks of blood glucose and plasma $K^+$
- Repeat as necessary
- *and/or* correction of severe acidosis (pH < 6.9): infuse $NaHCO_3$ (1.26%)
- *and/or* salbutamol 0.5 mg in 100 mL of 5% glucose over 15 min (rarely used)

**2. Later**
**Deplete body $K^+$ (to decrease plasma $K^+$ over the next 24 h):**
- Polystyrene sulphonate resins:
  - 15 g orally up to three times daily with laxatives
  - 30 g rectally followed 3–6 hours later by an enema
- Haemodialysis or peritoneal dialysis if the above fails

**Answer 13**
Initially, there is stimulation of the respiratory centre with hyperventilation leading to respiratory alkalosis. Metabolic acidosis ensues because of compensatory mechanisms including the renal excretion of bicarbonate and potassium as well as the accumulation of lactate, pyruvate and ketone bodies.

**Answer 14**
Bendroflumethiazide is a cheap, effective agent that, if given early in the day, causes a diuresis that does not interfere with sleep. Chlortalidone, another thiazide, has a longer action and can be given on alternate days. It is useful if a patient has prostatic symptoms as it produces a slower diuresis. Loop diuretics, e.g. furosemide and bumetanide, act within 1 hour of administration and would be used as first line in a severe acute situation, e.g. pulmonary oedema.

# 13 Cardiovascular disease

## QUESTIONS

### Question 1
What is the Bernheim effect and the reverse Bernheim effect?

### Question 2
Kindly explain why the left side of the heart is more prone to disease.

### Question 3
1. Is it always necessary to examine the cardiovascular system of a patient in the 45° incline of the head end? Other than convenience for examining the jugular venous pressure (JVP), does this position have any other advantage?
2. If the JVP is not visible when the patient is in the upright position, can one presume it is not raised?

### Question 4
The mitral area (of auscultation) normally corresponds with the apex beat. When the heart is dilated and the apex beat is shifted laterally, will the mitral area follow the apex beat to its new location or remain at the place where the apex beat is normally situated?

### Question 5
Please explain in detail how to measure the pulsus paradoxus using a sphygmomanometer.

### Question 6
What is the difference between dicrotic pulse and pulsus bisferiens?

### Question 7
1. Why does the radial pulse become more prominent when the hand is lifted overhead?

2. Please explain the mechanism of a collapsing pulse. Which is the best artery to elicit it: radial, brachial or carotid?

## Question 8
What is the mechanism of Durozier's sign?

## Question 9
What effects do aortic stenosis, aortic regurgitation and coarctation of the aorta have on systolic and diastolic blood pressure, and why do they produce these effects?

## Question 10
In the section headed 'Pulsus bisferiens' (K&C 6e, p. 736) what do 'percussion wave' and 'tidal wave' mean? An illustration here would be helpful.

## Question 11
When examining a patient's carotid pulse, why should we not palpate both carotids at once? Is it because it might block the blood supply to the brain?

## Question 12
How can I differentiate between jugular and arterial pulsation in the neck practically?

## Question 13
Can you please help me with this: 'Thrusting due to mitral or aortic regurgitation. Heaving due to aortic stenosis and systemic hypertension. There is often confusion about the terms thrusting and heaving'.

Another book I read considers aortic stenosis and hypertension for thrusting and mitral/aortic regurgitation for heaving. Who should I go with? Thank you.

## Question 14
Where is the best place on the precordium to auscultate a split-second heart sound?

## Question 15
What is the mechanism by which murmurs of mitral valve prolapse (MVP) and hypertrophic cardiomyopathy (HC) are accentuated by standing or the Valsalva manoeuvre?

## Question 16
What is the correct procedure for a fluoroscopy and why is this essential for the insertion of cardiac catheter, pacemaker and prosthetic valve?

## Question 17
What is the role of amiodarone in the acute management of asystole or pulseless electrical activity (PEA)?

## Question 18
1. Is there any contraindication to the use of microwaves or mobile phones in patients with pacemakers?
2. What, if any, appliances should be avoided in a patient with a pacemaker?

## Question 19
1. What is tachy-brady arrhythmia in the sick sinus syndrome?
2. How can it be managed?

## Question 20
Practically, how can we differentiate between a second-degree atrioventricular (AV) block Mobitz I and Mobitz II? What is the meaning of first-degree block? What is the difference between heart asystole, heart arrest and third-degree AV block?

## Question 21
How can a complete atrioventricular (AV) block be diagnosed on an electrocardiogram (ECG)?

## Question 22
Usually, we look for an R'SR pattern for bundle branch block in the chest leads. What does it mean if there is an R'SR pattern in the limb leads?

## Question 23
What is Wolff–Parkinson–White syndrome?

## Question 24
In management of atrial fibrillation (AF), is the priority to control ventricular rate or to restore cardiac rhythm?

## Question 25
Can digoxin be given in paroxysmal atrial fibrillation?

## Question 26
In a patient with atrial fibrillation and bronchial asthma, what is the recommended treatment and do beta-blockers make the condition worse?

## Question 27
What is the difference between atrial flutter and atrial tachycardia?

## Question 28
What are the possible causes of atrial extrasystoles, in a patient with a normal echo, which last for several days and then disappear spontaneously? Is treatment with anxiolytics recommended?

## Question 29
In the treatment of ventricular tachycardia, could lidocaine be used in the absence of any other drug? How effective is lidocaine?

## Question 30
Why is an extremely low level of potassium in the blood sometimes a cause of ventricular fibrillation?

## Question 31
How often does verapamil cause impotence and inhibit ejaculation?

## Question 32
Why does a patient with congestive cardiac failure have excessive sweating?

## Question 33
What is cardiac asthma?

## Question 34
In a book, under the title 'Heart failure' I have seen the following phrase: 'Cardiac failure occurs when, despite normal venous pressures, the heart is unable to maintain sufficient cardiac output…'. Is it correct to say 'normal venous pressures'? All protective and compensatory mechanisms raise the venous pressure to maintain a sufficient cardiac output – according to Frank–Starling law – and this is the case in heart failure, so I think it was meant to say: '…despite *high* venous pressures…'.

## Question 35
I wanted to ask whether a third heart sound is present, or should be present, in all cases of heart failure, whatever the underlying cause.

## Question 36
Why can left heart failure lead to right heart failure but not vice versa? What is the physiology involved in this transition?

## Question 37
Could you explain the fetal gene program, activated in heart failure?

## Question 38
How safe is it to stop administration of carvedilol to a patient with heart failure? Can the drug be tapered off? What are the effects/dangers of

stopping carvedilol suddenly? What, if any, are the reasons for discontinuing carvedilol in patients with heart failure?

## Question 39

What are the advantages and disadvantages of furosemide in the treatment of cardiac failure?

## Question 40

In heart failure, can furosemide be given once daily?

## Question 41

What are the clinical features of a ruptured sinus of Valsalva?

## Question 42

Does dobutamine (dose range 2.5–10 µg/kg/min) cause significant tachycardia?

## Question 43

Are beta-blockers indicated in heart failure; if yes, in all cases or in selected cases?

## Question 44

Why does long-term treatment by digitalis cause gynaecomastia?

## Question 45

Why do toxic doses of digoxin (which cause a decrease in excitability of cardiac tissue) cause arrhythmias, whereas therapeutic levels of digoxin (which cause increase in excitability) cause no arrhythmias?

## Question 46

Hypokalaemia is one of the complications of digitalis. In treatment we give $K^+$. How does the hyperkalaemia enhance the digitalis toxicity?

## Question 47

Why should we measure serum potassium before we start digoxin?

## Question 48

You state (*K&C 6e, p. 791*) that: 'The intravenous administration of loop diuretics such as furosemide relieves pulmonary oedema rapidly by means of arteriolar vasodilatation reducing afterload, an action that is independent of its diuretic effect'. However, I have been told that this drug has no effect on arterioles (except on efferent arterioles of the kidney), but rather a venodilatatory effect. What could be the cause of such different opinions?

## Question 49
There have been a number of recent publications concerning aspirin versus warfarin trials. Would you recommend prescribing warfarin for secondary prevention of coronary heart disease in patients suffering from their first myocardial infarction (MI)?

## Question 50
Is it true that in future the ApoA : ApoB ratio will be used to predict the risk of coronary artery disease more efficiently than low-density lipoprotein (LDL)?

## Question 51
What is the exact link between C-reactive protein (CRP) and coronary artery disease?

## Question 52
In angina pectoris, why does the chest pain get radiated to the left side, i.e. left arm and back?

## Question 53
Please explain why thrombolytic therapy is not indicated in cases of unstable angina and non-ST-segment elevation myocardial infarctions (nSTE-MI) despite the fact that both nSTE-MI and ST-elevated MI (STEMI) are caused by a thrombus for which thrombolytic therapy is highly indicated? Could it be true that, in the case of unstable angina and nSTE-MI has a higher incidence of intracranial haemorrhage than in the case of ST-segment elevation MI?

## Question 54
Doesn't the term 'acute coronary syndrome' include unstable angina, non-ST-segment elevation myocardial infarctions and ST-elevated MI (STEMI)?

## Question 55
Kindly mention the indications for clopidogrel in acute coronary syndrome (ACS). Should it be used along with aspirin or alone if the latter is contraindicated? Are there any studies that combine both with either low-molecular-weight heparin (LMWH) or unfractionated heparin? How long should clopidogrel be continued?

## Question 56
What role do IV fluids play in the management of acute inferior wall myocardial infarction?

## Question 57
Is there any benefit in combining aspirin with clopidogrel in post-MI angina and ischaemic stroke? A MATCH trial showed this combination

not to be of benefit – would you therefore recommend we stop using this combination in our hospital unit?

## Question 58
In a patient with the typical chest pain of myocardial infarction (MI) and no other criteria for thrombolysis would highly elevated cardiac enzymes indicate thrombolysis?

## Question 59
I cannot figure out the role of an acetylcholinesterase inhibitor in post-myocardial infarction from *Conn's Current Therapy* and *Swanson's Family Practice*. Can you help?

## Question 60
Can thrombolytic therapy for myocardial infarction (MI) be started in patients who have cardiac pain and raised cardiac markers? Can streptokinase be given irrespective of electrocardiogram (ECG) changes (according to some books, ST elevation has to be present)?

## Question 61
Can carvedilol be used in an elderly patient who developed left ventricular failure after a very recent myocardial infarction, or should it wait until the condition becomes stable?

## Question 62
I have seen some patients with chronic rheumatic heart disease with no obvious evidence of rheumatic fever (i.e. they could not recall if there was an episode of severe infection with subsequent fever and joint pain). So, actually, how is chronic rheumatic heart disease diagnosed?

## Question 63
If a young patient presents with hemiparesis and rheumatic atrial fibrillation and is already on oral anticoagulant, with an international normalized ratio (INR) = 3 and a normal computed tomography (CT) scan done 2 hours after onset, should he receive heparin for prophylaxis against further embolism? Should aspirin be combined with oral anticoagulant later, or should target INR be increased?

## Question 64
When treating mitral stenosis using a balloon valvotomy, how come no thrombus develops at the site of the atrial septum or at the separated commissure of the valve leaflets?

## Question 65
Why does a mitral stenosis produce a loud S1?

## Question 66
Why is the mitral valve more affected than any other valve in the heart in most valvular diseases?

## Question 67
What is William's syndrome (supravalvular obstruction)? Why does hypercalcaemia occur with this syndrome?

## Question 68
Kindly tell me all the causes postulated for the collapsing pulse seen in aortic regurgitation.

## Question 69
Does pulmonary stenosis cause pulmonary hypertension?

## Question 70
Under what conditions would a pulsatile liver be found and what is its clinical significance?

## Question 71
Can we use warfarin during pregnancy or during menstruation in a patient with a prosthetic valve? Is anticoagulation necessary in a patient with a corrected ventricular septal defect (VSD) or corrected coarctation of aorta?

## Question 72
I want to ask about Duke criteria in diagnosing infective endocarditis.

## Question 73
Is *Staphylococcus aureus* the most frequent causative agent of acute bacterial endocarditis? And is this typical of acute bacterial endocarditis?

## Question 74
Please explain the mechanism of the mycotic aneurysm in infective endocarditis.

## Question 75
Why are the right valves more commonly affected in infective endocarditis when the microbes enter through the IV route, for example with IV drug users?

## Question 76
You have said that in IV drug users the microbes go directly to the right ventricle, thus causing endocarditis in the right heart. But in dental

procedures the microbes also go through the veins to the right heart first, so why are the left heart valves more commonly affected?

## Question 77
What causes splenomegaly in infective endocarditis?

## Question 78
We know that Janeway lesions appear with infective endocarditis, but is there any other disease that can cause it?

## Question 79
Patent ductus arteriosus (PDA) is also called duct-dependent circulation. What is the meaning of this phrase and do any other conditions present with a similar condition? What is the implication of this condition to the human body?

## Question 80
What is the recommended treatment for a child with both congenital and valvular heart disease?

## Question 81
Can you describe a few instances that might cause a case of tetralogy of Fallot to go into congestive cardiac failure, even though this is an unlikely occurrence? Please explain how this happens.

## Question 82
Is a single ventricle disease associated with any syndrome? If so, what is its name and what are its characteristics?

## Question 83
What is the cause of splitting of the second sound in breathing and why is it wide and fixed in atrial septal defect (ASD)?

## Question 84
Why are deep-sea divers considered a 'high-risk' group if they have an atrial septal defect (ASD)?

## Question 85
Is it prognostically beneficial to start treatment of impending cor pulmonale in a case of chronic obstructive pulmonary disease (COPD) with no symptoms of failing heart but with investigational evidence (electrocardiogram and chest X-rays)?

## Question 86
What would be the ideal investigation for a suspected pulmonary embolism according to the protocol in a UK hospital?

## Question 87
Can the apical pulsation in right ventricular enlargement be hyperdynamic?

## Question 88
Please explain concentric and eccentric left ventricular hypertrophy. When the hypertrophied ventricle dilates and the wall thins out, is it still called a hypertrophied ventricle?

## Question 89
What is viral pericarditis?

## Question 90
I want to know why thrombolytic therapy is contraindicated in acute pericarditis.

## Question 91
Why would sitting bring pain relief to, and lying aggravate, a patient with acute pericarditis?

## Question 92
How do you determine whether a patient is in a 'hypertensive condition'? And what is wide pulse pressure?

## Question 93
I have a question about hypertension. Every textbook that I've come across places the greatest emphasis on the systolic blood pressure; it seems that diastolic pressure is often a figure that 'just happens to be there'. My question is: What is the clinical importance of a diastolic pressure? And what problems might arise if a patient has a too high/low diastolic blood pressure?

## Question 94
What causes hypertension in children?

## Question 95
Is haemochromatosis a cause of hypertension?

## Question 96
What are the most recent advancements in management of hypertensive crisis? Is there any new approach or method under trial?

## Question 97
Why does hypertension not cause headache, and why does only the accelerated hypertension cause headaches. You say in 'coarctation of aorta' that there is headache and epistaxis from hypertension.

## Question 98
Why is a headache one of the signs and symptoms of hypertension?

## Question 99
In a hypertensive hypercholesterolaemic patient, is it contraindicated to use a bisoprolol–hydrochlorothiazide combination to control the patient's hypertension if it is not controlled on bisoprolol alone?

## Question 100
Should a hypertensive patient with recurrent ischaemic strokes, a total cholesterol of 200 mg/dL (5.2 mmol/L), low-density lipoprotein (LDL) cholesterol of 120 mg/dL (3.12 mmol/L) and high-density lipoprotein (HDL) cholesterol of 35 mg/dL (<1 mmol/L), have a statin therapy?

## Question 101
Has Tenormin any advantage over other beta-blockers in the control of hypertension?

## Question 102
Is the use of sublingual captopril 25 mg/h, in combination with IV furosemide 40 mg/h to a maximum of 120 mg, safe to lower greatly elevated blood pressure?

## Question 103
Is ACEI superior to calcium channel blockers in the treatment of hypertension, in terms of prognosis and of the prevention of complications?

## Question 104
Are angiotensin-converting enzyme (ACE) inhibitors more effective than beta-blockers in reducing the risk of stroke in hypertensive patients?

## Question 105
Do non-steroidal anti-inflammatory drugs (NSAIDs) affect the antihypertensive effect of angiotensin-converting enzyme (ACE) inhibitors? If so, how?

## Question 106
What antihypertensive is recommended for a patient with aortic stenosis (AS) and hypertension, as a mono- and combination therapy?

## Question 107
Impotence is a common side-effect of antihypertensive drugs. How can I solve this problem in young hypertensive patients?

## Question 108

In the treatment of hypertension, is it recommended to commence treatment with two drugs containing a thiazide (if elderly) or a beta-blocker (if young)?

## Question 109

1. Following a stroke, both haemorrhagic and ischaemic, in previously hypertensive and normotensive patients, can you explain precise blood pressure control and the desired blood pressure levels?
2. In the case of a hypertensive emergency, with a blood pressure of 220/130 with acute myocardial infarction, what immediate measures should be taken?

## Question 110

On lowering blood pressure, to what extent can heart failure secondary to chronic hypertensive heart disease be reversible?

## Question 111

Is the use of amlodipine or furosemide recommended to normalize blood pressure in a case of hypertensive heart failure? If so, which is most effective?

## Question 112

How can diabetes cause endothelial dysfunction? What are the roles of ACE inhibitors in the kinin–kallikrein system? What are the mechanisms by which a decrease in the level of nitric oxide causes endothelial dysfunction?

## Question 113

Can sublingual nifedipine be given to a patient with malignant hypertension/accelerated hypertension? It seems to be a controversial issue with some favouring it and some against it.

## Question 114

Is the diagnosis of malignant hypertension based only on the basis of the retinopathy (even in the presence of a normotensive state)? Labetalol, parenterally, is suggested as a treatment for malignant hypertension. What other more readily available preparations (besides sodium nitroprusside) are recommended in addition to this drug? Parental labetalol is not available in Pakistan!

## Question 115

Patients at medium risk of DVT and pulmonary embolism are usually given specific prophylaxis with low-dose heparin at a dose of 5000 units subcutaneously every 8–12 hours until the patient is ambulatory. Is the first dose given *immediately* after, say, extensive varicose vein surgery of small and great saphenous veins?

### Question 116
'Anticoagulants are not necessary, as embolism does not occur from superficial thrombophlebitis' *(K&C 6e, p. 870)*. Why?

### Question 117
Can we use enoxaparin for deep vein thrombosis (DVT) prophylaxis in the immediate postoperative period and in a case of cerebral haemorrhage? Wouldn't it increase the risk of haemorrhage in either case?

### Question 118
Can external jugular vein thrombosis cause tingling numbness over the earlobe and adjoining part of the lower face?

### Question 119
For how long does a patient have to stay in bed to be labelled as bedridden and to merit low-molecular-weight heparin (LMWH) as prophylaxis for deep vein thrombosis?

### Question 120
Is an inferior vena cava filter an alternative treatment for a patient with a history of recurrent deep vein thrombosis on lifelong anticoagulation with warfarin?

### Question 121
Can you explain why a decrease in serum lipid levels follows an acute myocardial infarction (MI)? For how long does this decrease last and how is it known whether the patient has hyperlipidaemia in such a case?

### Question 122
In patients with myocardial infarction, why is aspirin to be taken chewed, and not by any other method?

## ANSWERS

### Answer 1

- The Bernheim effect: under normal circumstances there is a slight displacement of the inner ventricular septum into the right ventricular cavity because of the higher pressures on the left side of the heart.
- The reverse Bernheim effect: occurs when there is right ventricular overload, when displacement of the intraventricular septum into the left ventricular cavity occurs.

### Answer 2

It is presumably related to thickness of the left ventricle and workload compared to the right side. Diseases such as hypertension much more frequently affect the left side.

### Answer 3

1. No, it is mainly done for convenience; the JVP is normally just visible at this angle. The top of the JVP must be seen and therefore the position is irrelevant.
2. Probably, unless it is very high and the top of the column is behind the right ear. The JVP is acting like a U tube and does not have to be measured at 45° because the measurement is a vertical one (normal 3–4 cm above the manubrium sternum). 45° is convenient in that the JVP should just be seen at this angle. Sitting the patient up can allow a very high venous pressure to be seen whereas lying the patient flat can allow a low venous pressure to become visible.

### Answer 4

The mitral area follows the apex beat, often into the axilla.

### Answer 5

The pulse pressure (the difference between systolic and diastolic blood pressure) falls during inspiration. If you blow up the sphygmomanometer cuff to roughly the mid-point between diastolic and systolic pressure, the mercury column can be seen to be moving and falling on inspiration; an exaggerated fall greater than 10 mmHg can be seen in pulsus paradoxus.

### Answer 6

Bisferiens is two systolic peaks, the percussion and tidal waves. In dicrotic pulse, the second peak is in diastole immediately after the second heart sound (Fig. 13.1).

(a) Normal

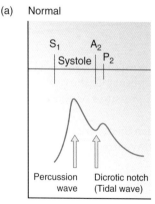

(b) Pulsus bisferiens

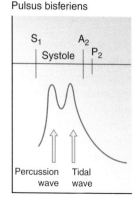

**Fig. 13.1** Configurational changes in the carotid pulse and their differential diagnosis. (a) Pulsus bisferiens, with percussion and tidal waves occurring during systole. This type of carotid pulse contour is observed most frequently in patients with dominant regurgitation; occasionally it is seen in patients with mitral valve prolpase or in normal individuals. (b) Dicrotic pulse. This results from an accentuated dicrotic wave and tends to occur in sepsis, severe heart failure, hypovolaemic shock, cardiac tamponade and after aortic valve replacement. $A_2$, aortic component of the second heart sound; $P_2$, pulmonary component of the second heart sound; $S_1$, first heart sound.

## Answer 7

1. Raising the arm does make the radial pulse easier to feel and this is more obvious with a large-volume pulse, which occurs in aortic regurgitation.
2. A collapsing pulse is due to an increased stroke volume, which gives quick distension of the peripheral arteries followed by regurgitation of blood back into the left ventricle, which gives a rapid fall, i.e. a quick rise followed by collapse. The brachial is probably the best artery to palpate.

## Answer 8

This is a femoral bruit ('pistol shot') due to a large volume pulse.

## Answer 9

Aortic stenosis can produce a low systolic pressure with a normal diastolic pressure because of outflow obstruction to the left ventricle (systolic) but normal peripheral resistance (diastolic). Aortic regurgitation produces normal or high systolic pressure because of unimpeded left ventricular emptying with low diastolic pressure due to a rapid fall in peripheral flow. Hypertension in coarctation is due to reduced renal flow (the Goldblatt effect).

## Answer 10
The percussion wave is the first wave produced by the transmission of the left ventricular pressure in early systole. With recoil of the vascular bed a second weaker wave (tidal) occurs which can be felt in the radial artery in the presence of slow ventricular emptying, e.g. in mixed aortic valve disease. A double pulse is bisferiens (Fig. 13.1).

## Answer 11
Yes, palpating each carotid separately is safer (one side may have a stenosis/atheroma) and might provide more information, e.g. right carotid sinus massage decreases the sinus node discharge. In addition, carotid sinus syncope can occur, which can impair cerebral perfusion in some elderly patients, causing loss of consciousness.

## Answer 12
- You can look for the double pulsation of the jugular venous pulse.
- You can feel the arterial pulse at the same time as you look at the jugular venous pulsation.
- The point at which the venous column is seen varies with the position of the patient.
- Pressure on the liver raises the jugular venous pressure, which can be used to make sure that it is the venous wave (hepato-jugular reflux).

## Answer 13
There is indeed confusion regarding the terms 'thrusting' and 'heaving'. We ourselves have changed the terms used to describe the apex beat over the six editions! You are also correct in saying that different terms are used by different authors. In the 6th edition we do not use the term 'thrusting'. Sustained (heaving) apex beat occurs in pressure overload situations, e.g. in aortic stenosis; forceful occurs with volume overload, e.g. aortic regurgitation.

## Answer 14
In the so-called pulmonary area: left substernal edge, second intercostal space.

## Answer 15
Standing or the 'strain phase' of the Valsalva manoeuvre decreases the left ventricular volume which increases the intensity and the duration of the murmur. 'Squatting' increases left ventricular volume and the murmur becomes shorter and softer.

## Answer 16
Fluoroscopy is dynamic radiography. X-rays are being taken continually so that the image is moving, not static as in a chest X-ray. Radiation

hazards limit the time used but it is invaluable in placing catheters etc. in the correct position.

## Answer 17

There is no role for amiodarone in asystole. Vasopressin does seem to be helpful.

*Further reading*

Wenzel V et al. (2004). A comparison of vasopressin and epinephrine for out-of-hospital cardiopulmonary resuscitation. *New England Journal of Medicine* **350**: 105–110.

## Answer 18

1. None with microwaves. Mobile phones should not be held right next to a pacemaker.
2. With modern pacemakers, no household appliances need to be avoided.

## Answer 19

1. In the sick sinus syndrome, patients develop episodes of sinus bradycardia or sinus arrest and commonly, owing to diffuse atrial disease, experience paroxysmal tachyarrhythmias. These together are called the tachy-brady syndrome.
2. A permanent pacemaker (paces the *A*trium, senses the *A*trium and *I*nhibits (AAI)) is required with antiarrhythmics to control the tachycardia element.

## Answer 20

Atrioventricular (AV) block is a block in either the AV node or in bundle of His, which means that impulses do not reach the ventricle during normal sinus rhythm or sinus tachycardia. The different types of block are seen on the ECG.

*First-degree AV block (Fig. 13.2a)*

This is prolongation of the PR interval to more than 0.22 s.

*Second-degree AV block*

- Type I, also called Mobitz type I or Wenckebach phenomenon (Fig. 13.2b): there is a progressive increase in the PR interval until a P wave fails to conduct.
- Type II or Mobitz type II (Fig. 13.2c): some P waves do not conduct to the ventricles and there is no progressive increase in the preceding complexes of the PR interval as in Mobitz type I.

*Third-degree AV block*

Complete heart block occurs when there is complete failure of conduction to the ventricles.

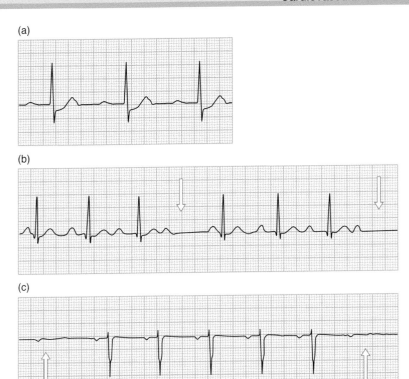

Fig. 13.2 (a) An electrocardiogram showing first-degree atrioventricular (AV) block with a prolonged PR interval. Coincidental ST depression is also present in this trace. (b) Wenckebach (Mobitz type I) AV block. The PR interval gradually prolongs until the P wave does not conduct to the ventricles (arrow). (c) Mobitz type II AV block. The P waves that do not conduct to the ventricles (arrow) are not preceded by gradual PR interval prolongation.

Cardiac arrest is sudden circulatory collapse due to the heart failing to pump blood from the ventricles. There are two mechanisms:
1. Ventricular fibrillation or ventricular tachycardia.
2. Asystole with no electrical activity of the ventricles.

### Answer 21
The ECG shows complete dissociation between the P wave and QRS complex (Fig. 13.3).

### Answer 22
This usually indicates a right bundle branch block with either right or left axis deviation, sometimes called a Wilson-type right bundle branch block.

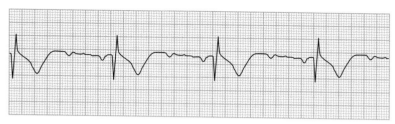

**Fig. 13.3** Acquired complete heart block. The QRS complex is broad (0.13 s) and the QRS rate is relatively slow (38 beats per minute).

## Answer 23

This describes patients with a history of palpitations in whom there is conduction down an accessory pathway producing a 'pre-excited' electrocardiogram. There is a short PR interval followed by a slurred initial part of the QRS complex known as the δ wave.

The electrical impulse is conducted quickly over the accessory pathway, thereby depolarizing the ventricle early, i.e. pre-excitation.

## Answer 24

There is greater emphasis at the present time in trying to control the rhythm, if this can be achieved, because anticoagulation can be stopped. This is discussed in Wyse et al. (2002).

*Reference*
Wyse DG, Waldo AL, DiMarco JP et al. (2002) A comparison of rate control and rhythm control in patients with atrial fibrillation. *New England Journal of Medicine* **347**: 1825–1833.

## Answer 25

Digoxin should not be used to prevent episodes of paroxysmal atrial fibrillation. Digoxin can be used to slow the heart rate in a patient who is in atrial fibrillation. The treatment of choice to prevent further attacks is by catheter ablation of the arrhythmic focus.

## Answer 26

The treatment is either cardioversion (rhythm control) or AV nodal slowing agents (rate control) but you need to carefully study the management of this common condition. Beta-blockers should not be used in patients with asthma; it makes the asthma worse.

## Answer 27

Atrial flutter is an organized atrial rhythm at 250–350 beats per minute. The most frequent is counterclockwise flutter, but re-entry flutter also occurs. Atrial tachycardia is slower and is either a re-entry or automatic tachycardia.

## Answer 28
Atrial ectopic beats are usually of no significance. Treatment is not usually required but a beta-blocker can be used, particularly with anxiety.

## Answer 29
Yes, lidocaine given as a bolus followed by intravenous infusion (2–4 mg/min) is very effective. DC cardioversion is the other option.

## Answer 30
Hypokalaemia affects repolarization with progressively smaller T waves. Usually, this has no immediate consequence but, particularly in the presence of digoxin, ventricular fibrillation can occur.

## Answer 31
This is unclear. Most people think all hypotensive agents can produce erectile dysfunction, but, in one study comparing a number of drugs only thiazides caused more dysfunction than placebo.

## Answer 32
Excessive sweating is related to increased circulating sympathomimetics such as epinephrine (adrenaline).

## Answer 33
Wheezing due to bronchial endothelial oedema occurs in cardiac failure and is sometimes called 'cardiac asthma' to compare and contrast it with bronchial asthma.

## Answer 34
Both normal or high venous pressure are correct. This phrase is used to exclude low pressure from hypoperfusion when the heart has not failed but there is still no cardiac output.

## Answer 35
Yes, it is present in left ventricular failure of whatever cause. The precise mechanism of the cause of the third heart sound is not entirely clear. It is associated with rapid ventricular filling.

## Answer 36
Left heart failure is much more common than right heart failure and in the backward pressure theory of heart failure right ventricular failure develops as a consequence of left ventricular failure.

## Answer 37
Changes in the myocardial gene expression occur when the ventricle is overloaded, i.e. heart failure and there is a return to the fetal pattern, as

shown in animal models. There is a shift from $\alpha\alpha$ (usually predominates in the atrium) to $\beta\beta$ (usually mainly in the ventricles) myosin heavy chains in the atria.

## Answer 38

There appear to be no dangers in stopping carvedilol suddenly or indeed tapering off the drug. However, most patients should not have the drug withdrawn, because of the good results reported with beta-blocker usage. In one small study in patients who were taken off a beta-blocker, deterioration or death occurred in 50% of a small group of patients. Finally, bradycardia and poor cardiac output are the usual reasons for discontinuing carvedilol and it is not appropriate to use it if a drug such as milrinone is being considered.

## Answer 39

Furosemide promotes renal excretion of water and sodium, so relieving fluid overload, i.e. oedema. It also has a venodilatory action, which is why pulmonary oedema responds rapidly to IV furosemide. Its main side-effect is hypokalaemia.

## Answer 40

Yes; usually 40 mg in the morning is given, to avoid nocturnal urinary frequency.

## Answer 41

This usually occurs in a previously fit young man who suddenly has shortness of breath and ischaemic chest pain. Heart failure is present with a loud continuous murmur on auscultation. Echocardiography is diagnostic. Treatment is urgent surgery.

## Answer 42

At this dosage there is an increase in myocardial contractility with little effect on rate.

## Answer 43

All patients with heart failure should receive a beta-blocker if there is no contraindication, e.g. asthma, and if the drug is tolerated (in clinical trials >85% of patients tolerated beta-blockers). The initial dose should be low to avoid initial side-effects, e.g. hypotension. In randomized controlled trials, beta-blockers have been shown to improve symptoms as well as reduce the risk of death and retard the progression of heart failure.

## Answer 44

Elevated plasma oestradiol levels (digoxin has intrinsic oestrogenic properties) and decreased plasma testosterone levels occur.

## Answer 45

Toxic levels of digoxin cause an increase in intracellular calcium, which leads to depolarization of the cells, initiating arrhythmia.

## Answer 46

Hypokalaemia is not a direct complication of digitalis therapy. Vomiting, anorexia and diarrhoea are side-effects of digoxin therapy and can contribute to hypokalaemia. Hyperkalaemia does not enhance digitalis toxicity but too rapid a correction of hypokalaemia can lead to heart block.

## Answer 47

Digoxin acts by inhibiting the $Na^+-K^+$-ATPase pump. Hypokalaemia increases the binding of digoxin to cardiac myocytes, potentiating its action and decreasing its clearance as well as further inhibiting the $Na^+-K^+$-ATPase pump. Hypokalaemia should be corrected (it should of course not be allowed to occur) in patients on digoxin. Paradoxically, hyperkalaemia can occur in severe digoxin overdose, and might need treatment with glucose and insulin.

## Answer 48

Loop diuretics do primarily act on venules producing an acute increase in systemic venous capacitance and thereby decreasing left ventricular filling pressure. This effect is probably mediated by prostaglandins released from the kidney. Some workers think that furosemide has an effect on arterioles similar to morphine in pulmonary oedema. We agree the text could be clearer!

## Answer 49

At the present time, aspirin is used routinely in all patients following an MI unless there are contraindications. Warfarin is used if there is evidence of a deep vein thrombosis (DVT), pulmonary embolism, mural thrombosis on an echocardiogram, the presence of atrial fibrillation or a previous embolic cardiovascular event.

## Answer 50

Apo A : Apo B ratio is not more effective for predicting coronary artery disease than LDL.

## Answer 51

CRP is an independent risk factor for coronary artery disease. Atherosclerosis is an inflammatory condition and CRP elevation may therefore occur. Recent data have, however, questioned whether CRP is in fact, an independent factor.

*Further reading*
Hansson GK (2005) Inflammation, atherosclerosis and coronary artery disease. *New England Journal of Medicine* **352**; 1685–1695 (review).

## Answer 52

Pain from the heart is transmitted by visceral afferent fibres accompanying sympathetic fibres and is typically referred to the upper chest and left arm, which have afferent fibres with cell bodies in the same spinal ganglion and central processes that enter the spinal cord through the same dorsal roots. The pain is typically felt in the area supplied by the medial cutaneous nerve of the arm (T1 spinal segment). Communicating fibres in the spinal cord to the right side explain the occurrence of pain that occurs in both arms or occasionally only in the right arm.

*Further reading*
Hardy SGP, Naftel JP (1996) Viscerosensory pathways. In: Haines DE (ed) *Fundamental Neuroscience*. New York: Churchill Livingstone.

## Answer 53

The terminology has changed slightly. STEMI still refers to ST segment elevation myocardial infarction but both non-ST elevation myocardial infarction and unstable angina are now referred to as nSTE-ACS (ACS being acute coronary syndrome).

Fibrinolytic agents are not used in nSTE-ACS because they do not reduce the mortality. Coronary intervention is now used for many cases in many institutions but the beneficial effects are still being studied.

*Further reading*
Stone GW (2007) Non-ST elevation acute coronary syndromes. *Lancet* **369**: 801–803.

## Answer 54

The term 'acute coronary syndrome' (ACS) was introduced to refer to unstable angina but now includes nSTE-ACS and STEMI as well as unstable angina (see above and McClelland et al. 2004). It is necessary, for optimal treatment, to stratify patients with acute coronary syndrome into high and low risk.

*Reference*
McClelland AJ et al. (2004) Acute coronary syndromes. *Clinical Medicine* **4**: 27–31.

## Answer 55

The CURE trial, which involved over 12 000 patients, compared treatment with aspirin and aspirin plus clopidogrel. There was some suggestion of a better outcome with the two drugs but there was an increase in haemorrhagic complications. It was therefore recommended that clopidogrel be used for those people in whom aspirin is contraindicated. However, current guidelines recommend that aspirin *and* clopidogrel should be given to all patients with acute coronary syndromes unless cardiac bypass surgery is planned. There have been no published studies on unfractionated heparin or low-molecular-weight heparin with clopidogrel. Finally, the clopidogrel should be continued for at least 9–12 months.

*Further reading*
Opie LH et al. (2006) Controversies in stable coronary artery disease. *Lancet* **367**: 64–78.

## Answer 56
Acute inferior wall infarction can be accompanied by right ventricular dysfunction, when hypotension might be present, with a low cardiac output and low venous pressure. A fluid challenge with 0.9% saline can be helpful, as volume expansion might be needed.

## Answer 57
Controversial! Long-term use of clopidogrel with aspirin increases the risk of bleeding without having much effect on outcome. However, the Scottish Medicine Consortium advised (in February 2004) that clopidogrel be accepted for restricted use with low-dose aspirin for non-ST elevation acute coronary syndrome (nSTE-ACS) and many authorities now use clopidogrel and aspirin in all patients with acute coronary syndrome. Not useful in ischaemic stroke.

## Answer 58
With chest pain and high troponins only non-ST elevation acute coronary syndrome (nSTE-ACS) is not usually considered an indication for thrombolysis. Views change and, as you know, coronary angiography and stenting seem to be replacing thrombolysis when available.

## Answer 59
Acetylcholinesterase inhibitors (i.e. antimuscarinics, which is a better term) such as atropine are used for sinus bradycardia following myocardial infarction.

## Answer 60
The use of thrombolytic therapy continually changes. The diagnosis of MI was also changed to include a classic history and raised troponins. More recently, however, streptokinase therapy or other thrombolytics have been recommended only for patients with ECG changes of ST elevation (STEMI) (Fig. 13.4). Non-STEMI (no ST elevation) patients are not given thrombolytic therapy, even though troponins are raised, but are referred for coronary angioplasty.

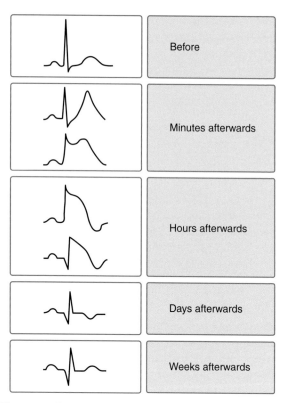

**Fig. 13.4** Electrocardiographic evolution of ST-elevated myocardial infarction (STEMI). After the first few minutes, the T waves become tall, pointed and upright and there is ST segment elevation. After the first few hours, the T waves invert, the R wave voltage is decreased and Q waves develop. After a few days, the ST segment returns to normal. After weeks or months the T wave might return to upright but the Q wave remains.

## Answer 61
Beta-blockers such as carvedilol have shown a significant improvement in the survival in patients with chronic *stable* heart failure. Therefore wait until the patient is stabilized with angiotensin-converting enzyme (ACE) inhibitor ± diuretics.

## Answer 62
Only 50% of patients with chronic rheumatic heart disease give a history of rheumatic fever or chorea. There is no absolute way one can be sure that the valvular disease is rheumatic – it is by exclusion of other causes, e.g. syphilis in aortic regurgitation. Mitral stenosis is almost always due to rheumatic fever.

## Answer 63

This is difficult, but there is no evidence that using another agent, e.g. heparin, helps. Aspirin has been used but efficacy is not very good. Consideration should be given to treatment of the valvular lesion, which will include removal of clot from the left atrium and then DC cardioversion or drug therapy to control the rhythm.

## Answer 64

It is unclear why this does not happen but it does not seem to! Percutaneous treatment using a balloon compares very favourably with open and closed valvotomy with no evidence of early or late thromboembolism in any group.

## Answer 65

The valve leaflets are widely open when ventricular systole begins and therefore they close with a loud noise.

## Answer 66

There is no good reason for this.

## Answer 67

Williams syndrome is a rare genetic syndrome that includes supravalvular alveolar aortic stenosis, narrowing of the pulmonary arteries and many other features.

It is unclear why hypercalcaemia occurs. There is no abnormality of parathyroid hormone (PTH) secretion and vitamin D levels are normal. An abnormality in the gene regulating calcitonin and calcitonin-gene-related peptide has been suggested.

## Answer 68

Rapid ejection of left ventricular volume into a low-resistance arterial system followed by regurgitation back into the left ventricle leads to a rapid fall in pressure with collapse of the arterial pressure.

## Answer 69

No, there is no significant rise in pulmonary pressure in most cases of pulmonary stenosis.

## Answer 70

A palpable liver that pulsates in systole is seen in a tricuspid regurgitation. It is associated with right heart failure.

## Answer 71

Warfarin is teratogenic and should not be given in the first trimester, and women at risk of pregnancy should be warned to stop the drug very early. The use of anticoagulation in pregnancy is a very complicated problem and should only be done under careful supervision by people expert in the field. Anticoagulation is not necessary for a corrected VSD or coarctation of the aorta.

## Answer 72

These are the clinical criteria described at Duke University, North Carolina, for the diagnosis of infective endocarditis (*see K&C 6e, p. 830*). The two major criteria are a positive blood culture and evidence of valvular disease, either clinical or echocardiographic. Minor criteria include fever, evidence of emboli, etc. Two major or one major and three minor are required for the diagnosis of infective endocarditis.

## Answer 73

*Staph. aureus* is the most common cause of acute bacterial endocarditis. The clinical picture is very typical.

## Answer 74

Small septic emboli block vasa vasorum or a small distal cerebral artery itself, leading to damage to the muscular layer with dilatation and aneurysm formation.

## Answer 75

Because a large number of organisms go directly to the valves on the right side. However, even in intravenous drug users, left-sided valve involvement is more common.

## Answer 76

It is a question of the amount of bacteria, which is large in IV drug users and small in dental sepsis. The reason for the left heart valves being affected more in, for example, dental procedures is probably because the incidence of damage to the left heart valves, e.g. from rheumatic fever, is greater than the right.

## Answer 77

This is probably due to chronic infection with stimulation of both humoral and cellular immunity.

## Answer 78

Janeway lesions are fairly specific for infective endocarditis.

## Answer 79

Duct-dependent circulation occurs in fetal life when there is no pulmonary circulation. The blood is diverted through the duct (that is, duct dependent) into the systemic circulation and is then re-oxygenated as it passes through the placenta. There is no comparable situation. Failure of ductal closure at birth results in persistent ductus arteriosus, which can lead to cardiac problems if not treated.

## Answer 80
Careful evaluation in a designated centre with echocardiography (including Doppler) and MRI is carried out initially. Corrective surgery is performed if necessary in a stepwise fashion.

## Answer 81
We cannot explain this rare complication.

## Answer 82
Single ventricle disease is where the blood flowing through the mitral and tricuspid valves enters one common ventricle, morphologically in 90% of cases it is the left ventricle. The effects are complex and most require surgery as a baby, with the formation of anastomoses between the systemic venous and pulmonary circulations.

## Answer 83
In inspiration left ventricular systole shortens causing A2 to occur earlier. In inspiration there is increased venous return to the right heart which further delays P2. Therefore the split in the second sound is wider. In an uncomplicated ASD, shunting of blood from the left to the right heart occurs, which counterbalances the normal respiratory variation in systemic venous return; therefore the split is fixed.

## Answer 84
Because paradoxical emboli occur with production of a stroke.

## Answer 85
Oxygen therapy given continuously has been shown to reduce pulmonary artery pressure, and to decrease mortality in COPD. Other agents to reduce pulmonary pressure, such as vasodilators, are probably of no benefit and may be harmful.

*Further reading*
Wiedemann HP, Matthay RA (1990) Cor pulmonale in chronic obstructive pulmonary disease. Circulatory pathophysiology and management. *Clinics in Chest Medicine* **11**: 525.

## Answer 86
Ventilation–perfusion scan. A normal scan virtually excludes a pulmonary embolism. A 'high probability' scan indicates a 95% chance of a pulmonary embolism. A negative D-dimer assay excludes a pulmonary embolism. All of these investigations must be evaluated with the clinical

features. If obtainable, a multi-slice CT has a high sensitivity even with a small embolus

*Further reading*
Stein P D et al. (2006) Multidetector computed tomography for acute pulmonary embolism. *New England Journal of Medicine* **354**: 2317.

## Answer 87
Not usually.

## Answer 88
Concentric hypertrophy occurs with hypertension; the left ventricular wall becomes uniformly thickened but the intraventricular end-diastolic volume remains unchanged. Eccentric hypertrophy occurs with mitral regurgitation; the end-diastolic volume is increased but wall thickness is not. In both, histologically and ultrastructurally, there is hypertrophy.

*Further reading*
Opie LH (2006) Ventricular remodelling. *Lancet* **367**: 356–367.

## Answer 89
Acute pericarditis (inflammation of the pericardium) is often due to a virus. Coxsackie and echovirus are the most common causes in the UK.

## Answer 90
Thrombolytic therapy is not required in acute pericarditis; there is no problem with the coronary arteries. Pericarditis complicating myocardial infarction is not a contraindication to thrombolytic therapy, although of course thrombolytic therapy should have been given long before pericarditis developed.

## Answer 91
Sitting forward in some way separates the chest wall fractionally from the parietal pericardium. There must be other local factors.

## Answer 92
Hypertension is defined as a systolic pressure above 130–139 and/or a diastolic blood pressure of 85–89 mmHg. Wide pulse pressure means an increase in the pressure between systolic and diastolic values. For example, normal pulse pressure in a patient with BP 120/70 = 50; wide pulse pressure in a patient with BP 160/60 = 100. This is common in the elderly with stiff, non-compliant arteries.

## Answer 93
The diastolic pressure is of critical value and until fairly recently was the main target of treatment. This was because the diastolic pressure does not

vary as much as the systolic and therefore clear guidance could be given that patients with a diastolic pressure > 100 mmHg should be treated; this value is now more usually > 90 mmHg. Recently, it has been realized that the systolic pressure is as important in the production of complications – both cerebrovascular and cardiac events.

Isolated systolic hypertension occurs frequently in the elderly > 160 mmHg and needs treatment (Table 13.1).

## Answer 94
Look for:
- renal disease
- endocrine disease
- coarctation of the aorta.

## Answer 95
No; haemochromatosis is not a cause of hypertension.

## Answer 96
The most recent advance in management reflects CT and MRI imaging, which show the effect of accelerated hypertension on the brain. In terms

**Table 13.1 British Hypertension Society classification of blood pressure levels**

| Category | Systolic blood pressure (mmHg) | Diastolic blood pressure (mmHg) |
|---|---|---|
| **Blood pressure** | | |
| Optimal | <120 | <80 |
| Normal | <130 | <85 |
| High normal | 130–139 | 85–89 |
| **Hypertension** | | |
| Grade 1 (mild) | 140–159 | 90–99 |
| Grade 2 (moderate) | 160–179 | 100–109 |
| Grade 3 (severe) | >180 | >110 |
| **Isolated systolic hypertension** | | |
| Grade 1 | 140–149 | <90 |
| Grade 2 | >160 | <90 |

The classification equates with those of the European Society of Hypertension and the World Health Organization International Society of Hypertension and is based on clinical blood pressure and not values for ambulatory blood pressure measurement. Threshold blood pressure levels for the diagnosis of hypertension using self/home monitoring are greater than 135/85 mmHg. For ambulatory monitoring, 24-h values are greater than 125/80 mmHg. If systolic blood pressure and diastolic blood pressure fall into different categories, the higher value should be taken for classification.

of treatment, the most important thing is not to reduce the pressure too quickly except in very urgent situations, e.g. a dissecting aneurysm. Here parenteral therapy is necessary. In other situations, oral hypotensive therapy only should be used. This can be with atenolol, labetalol or a calcium-channel blocker, e.g. amlodipine. Try to reduce pressure over 24 hours to between 100 and 110 mmHg diastolic.

## Answer 97
Hypertension does not normally cause headache. Accelerated hypertension does cause headaches because there is some degree of cerebral oedema. In a number of descriptions of coarctation of the aorta it does say that headache and epistaxis is a clinical feature; there is no good explanation for this headache.

## Answer 98
Headache only occurs with severe hypertension where there are associated changes in the small cerebral arteries.

## Answer 99
No, the combination is not contraindicated as it is an effective treatment of hypertension although recent guidelines do not recommend beta-blockers. It is true that thiazide and beta-blocker therapy does affect the cholesterol but the change is usually small and if necessary a statin can be co-prescribed.

## Answer 100
Total cholesterol <200 mg/dL (5.2 mmol/L) is desirable with an LDL cholesterol <100 mg/dL. The HDL cholesterol should be greater than 60 mg/dL (>1.5 mmol/L). So, yes, statin therapy is required, with lifestyle changes.

## Answer 101
Tenormin (atenolol) is the most commonly prescribed beta-blocker for hypertension. It is water soluble, and therefore has no effect on the brain. It has no other advantage, except that it is cheap. Recent data suggest that atenolol only reduces the brachial and not aortic pressure and therefore has no effect on outcome.

### Further reading
Wilkinson IB et al. (2006) Atenolol and cardiovascular risk; an issue close to the heart. *Lancet* **367**: 627–629.

## Answer 102
We have not used this combination. Captopril is almost always used orally not sublingually. 'Do not reduce the blood pressure too rapidly' is the rule, even when the initial readings are very high.

## Answer 103

ACE inhibitors are thought to be the drug of choice for hypertension in the diabetic as they are renoprotective. Both reduce the risk of stroke. Often both drugs are needed for good control of hypertension. In non-diabetics, both are useful.

*Further reading*
Kaplan NM, Opie LH (2006) Controversies in hypertension. *Lancet* **367**: 168–176.

## Answer 104

No. Beta-blockers are still as effective as the newer agents such as ACE inhibitors, although the new drugs are being more and more used because side-effects are less. ACE inhibitors or ACE antagonists are recommended in diabetics.

*Further reading*
Williams B (2006) Evolution of hypertensive disease: a revolution in guidelines. *Lancet* **368**: 6–8.

## Answer 105

Yes. They promote $Na^+$ retention and have an effect on prostaglandin synthesis in the kidney.

## Answer 106

If the patient is asymptomatic no treatment is required for aortic stenosis (AS). Hypertension could be treated with beta-blockers. Surgery is usually indicated in patients with symptoms from AS. Hypertension could be treated with a diuretic plus beta-blockers with careful evaluation.

## Answer 107

Impotence (a better term is erectile dysfunction) is common with antihypertensive therapy. Try to avoid drugs such as bendroflumethiazide, which is well recognized as causing erectile dysfunction. Fortunately, most patients respond to phosphodiesterase type 5 inhibitors (PDE5), e.g. sildenafil, even on hypotensive therapy.

## Answer 108

It is usual to start with a single agent, although this is often not adequate and a second agent is required. Conventional treatment is to start with a thiazide diuretic, then adding a beta-blocker as you suggest. Many doctors now, however, go straight to an angiotensin-converting enzyme inhibitor or ACE blocker, which tend to have a better side-effect profile. Also, calcium-channel blocking drugs are often used.

## Answer 109

1. Control of blood pressure is of vital importance but should not be achieved rapidly. Oral therapy, e.g. amlodipine, is used to bring the

diastolic pressure to below 100 mmHg initially. Longer-term combination therapy is usually required to get blood pressure to 120 systolic, 80 diastolic, ideally.

2. In the patient with a myocardial infarction the same principles apply: use oral medication to get the diastolic pressure down to 100–110 mmHg over 24 hours.

## Answer 110
Controlling hypertension in the elderly can reduce the incidence of heart failure by 30%. Heart failure is reversible but still carries a high mortality.

## Answer 111
Both can be used and dual or triple therapy is often required in hypertension.

## Answer 112
Diabetes is associated with atherosclerosis, which causes endothelial dysfunction (Gaenzer et al. 2002). ACE inhibitors inhibit the inactivation of bradykinin and substance P. Nitric oxide causes vasodilatation so that any decrease in nitric oxide promotes constriction and therefore endothelial damage.

*Reference*
Gaenzer H et al. (2002) Effect of insulin therapy on endothelium-dependent dilation in type 2 diabetes mellitus. *American Journal of Cardiology* **89**: 431.

## Answer 113
Sublingual nifedipine is recommended by some authorities for malignant hypertension and therefore you can give it. The main aim is not to lower the blood pressure too rapidly. You are best to use the agent that you are familiar with. Other agents include atenolol or amlodipine but sublingual modified-release nifedipine is quite acceptable.

## Answer 114
To diagnose *hyper*tension you must have a raised blood pressure. Malignant hypertension is associated with grade 3–4 retinopathy.

Malignant hypertension should always be treated with oral medication if possible. Parenteral therapy might be required if there are complications; parenteral nitroprusside is the preferred agent but requires careful monitoring. Intravenous diazoxide, oral clonidine and oral nifedipine are used when labetalol is not available.

## Answer 115
Many experts now advocate preoperative treatment (e.g. 2 hours before surgery) in medium- and high-risk patients. Many clinicians now use low-molecular-weight heparin, e.g. enoxaparin 40 mg, rather than

low-dose unfractionated heparin. *Note*: other prophylactic techniques, e.g. compression stockings, should also be used.

## Answer 116
There is inflammation of the vein wall so that the thrombus adheres to it and pulmonary embolism occurs only rarely.

## Answer 117
No, it should not be used in a case of cerebral haemorrhage. Enoxaparin, a low-molecular-weight heparin, is used quite safely without monitoring in DVT prophylaxis postoperatively.

## Answer 118
This seems very unlikely.

## Answer 119
This depends partly on risk factors such as age, obesity, degree of immobilization and how long the period in bed is likely to be. Medical patients are sometimes not treated with LMWH as early as they should be, partly because there are no clear guidelines. Treat early, if possible, with LMWH. Guidelines are available for surgical patients.

*Further reading*
Guidelines on oral anticoagulation (1990) *British Journal of Haematology* **101**: 704–715.

## Answer 120
Filters in the inferior vena cava are useful for preventing recurrent pulmonary emboli rather than using long-term warfarin. Anticoagulation can be stopped with a filter in place.

## Answer 121
The decrease in lipid levels is related to increased adrenalin which affects lipid levels for up to 3 months. It doesn't occur for 24–36 hours so there is usually time for samples to be taken. Otherwise, you will have to wait 3 months to confirm hyperlipidaemia, unless of course the serum lipids are *high* after the MI.

## Answer 122
Aspirin chewed goes directly into the systemic circulation; if you swallow it, it has to be absorbed in the gut and then be transported by the portal system.

# 14 Respiratory disease

## QUESTIONS

### Question 1
As a third-year medical student in Russia I am researching 'the role of proteolytic enzymes and their inhibitors in lung pathology'. Can you explain how proteolytic enzymes function in the normal lung?

### Question 2
Bronchiectasis is given as one of the causes of bronchial breath sounds. This is difficult to comprehend. Could you explain the mechanism of bronchial breath sounds more clearly?

### Question 3
I have been taught to examine vocal resonance by asking the patient to say 'ninety-nine' while auscultating. I listen for a louder 'ninety-nine' over an area of consolidation and more quiet sounds with effusion. Is this right?

### Question 4
What role does bupropion play in giving up smoking?

### Question 5
The clinical signs and symptoms of rhinitis are very similar to those of the common cold (influenza). How do I differentiate between the two?

### Question 6
What is the advantage of the drugs des-loratidine and levo-cetirizine over their parent compounds? Are they safe in pregnancy and lactation?

### Question 7
What are the differences between acute bronchitis and pneumonia? Are both diseases caused by infection?

## Question 8

1. If a patient with chronic bronchitis develops obstructive jaundice and *Escherichia coli* biliary sepsis, should the routine administration of oral steroids (e.g. prednisolone) be suspended until liver function improves?

2. Are there any adverse reactions that preclude the concurrent use of steroids while the patient is treated with IV ciprofloxacin, gentamicin, metronidazole and cefuroxime?

## Question 9

*Robbins Basic Pathology* mentions that in patients with chronic obstructive pulmonary disease (COPD), the forced ventilation capacity (FVC) is either normal or slightly increased! I just can't justify that. I mean it should decrease. And this is exactly what is mentioned in your book. I couldn't contact the authors of that book so I decided to ask you whether there is actually a situation in which the FVC in COPD patients might increase?

## Question 10

Is there any obstructive pulmonary condition in which there might be an increase in FVC? If so by what mechanism?

## Question 11

I am confused whether clubbing is a feature of chronic obstructive pulmonary disease (COPD) or not – you have mentioned that it is not a feature of COPD but some books do say that clubbing is a clinical feature of COPD.

## Question 12

A 70-year-old man with chronic obstructive pulmonary disease (COPD) and a past history of myocardial infarction with a left ventricular ejection fraction (LVEF) of 25% is dyspnoeic on slight exertion such as walking, bathing. He is not orthopnoeic and claims to have no paroxysmal nocturnal dyspnoea (PND). He has no wheezing or productive cough and his blood pressure is normal. He has had three episodes of ventricular tachycardia (VT) and has been on amiodarone for the past year. What is the best way to determine the exact cause of dyspnoea in this case?

## Question 13

In bronchiectasis, what is the reason for using a bronchodilator if the airways are already dilated?

## Question 14

Why is it that asthmatics having a severe attack can be seen clawing their hands?

## Question 15
Practical use of steroids:
- Which form of regimen is better (alternate-day, daily or in pulse form)?
- What should be the dose (once daily or three times daily or {2/3} in the morning)?
- For how long, especially when to give short courses as in asthmatics, when we don't need to taper it down?

## Question 16
In pregnancy, what is the recommended treatment for bronchial asthma? Is the use of the long-acting beta-adrenergic agonist Seretide, the corticosteroid Symbicort and leucotriene receptor antagonists (LTRAs) recommended?

## Question 17
In asthma patients, which is the safest analgesic to use?

## Question 18
Is the use of nebulized heparin in the treatment of asthmatic attacks recommended?

## Question 19
I would like to ask you about pneumonia and its classifications in particular; what are they?

## Question 20
What are the pathological differences in typical and atypical pneumonia?

## Question 21
Why, sometimes in cases of aspiration pneumonia, would the level of lymphocytes drop below normal range while the level of white blood cells (WBC) and neutrophils are above normal range?

## Question 22
Should steroids be used in the treatment of a standard case of pneumonia in a young child?

## Question 23
I want to know more about the epidemiology and pathophysiology of this severe acute respiratory syndrome (SARS) scare and what advances have been made in its therapy.

## Question 24
What symptoms will confirm, without doubt, a diagnosis of tuberculosis?

## Question 25
Please could you tell me the skin-prick test result for non-infected and non-immune tuberculosis carriers?

## Question 26
Please can you help me find the answer to whether the purified protein derivative (PPD) in the tuberculin skin test develops memory T lymphocytes? If so, would it not be confusing with the way BCG vaccine works?

## Question 27
In diseases that have night sweats as a symptom (e.g. tuberculosis, infective endocarditis), what causes the sweats to occur only at night and not consistently during the day as well?

## Question 28
An asymptomatic patient, whose tuberculous pleural effusion has subsided after a year's treatment of anti-TB, is left with a small loculated effusion, apparent on ultrasound and chest X-ray. Should this be aspirated?

## Question 29
I want to know what are the exact indications for using steroids in patients with tuberculous pleural effusions/ascites?

## Question 30
Should prednisolone be added to the anti-tuberculosis therapy in all cases of massive tuberculous effusion? Does the quick absorption help prevent fibrosis?

## Question 31
In the case of antituberculous treatment toxicity, how high should the serum glutamic pyruvate transaminase (SGPT) rise before we should stop treatment?

## Question 32
After starting antituberculous treatment, when is the fever expected to subside and the erythrocyte sedimentation rate (ESR) to return to normal?

## Question 33
What are the indications of steroids in the treatment of tuberculosis?

## Question 34
I am a final-year medical student in India, where tuberculosis in all forms is one of the most common diseases with which we deal. I read that you feel there is no indication for steroids in tuberculosis. Is it not reasonable

to give steroids with antitubercular therapy (ATT) in a patient with tuberculous pericarditis, meningitis, peritonitis and ocular manifestations due to tuberculosis, in order to reduce the damage caused by inflammation and fibrosis? If not, what suitable alternatives, other than steroids, would you recommend to reduce damage from postinflammatory fibrosis?

## Question 35
What dosage of steroids and duration of treatment should be given to patients with idiopathic pulmonary fibrosis? What are the new drugs, their recommended dosage and duration of treatment?

## Question 36
What is the poor prognostic factor in cryptogenic fibrosis: fibrosis or concomitant connective tissue disorder?

## Question 37
Are wheezes present in extrinsic allergic alveolitis?

## Question 38
Is the measurement of chest expansion with a tape a useful physical examination to indicate the severity of emphysema?

## Question 39
In asbestos-related pleural disease (pleural plaques and mesothelioma), how do asbestos fibres get to the pleural space?

## Question 40
How do you differentiate clinically between thickened pleura and pleural effusion?

## Question 41
What is the difference between transudate and exudate?

## Question 42
I wish to ask about Meigs' syndrome. I know that it is an association of pleural effusion, ascites and benign ovarian tumours or fibromas. Is the effusion transudate or exudate?

## Question 43
I have read that patients with cystic fibrosis should not meet each other socially. Why is this?

## Question 44
I have a young patient with bilateral hilar lymphadenopathy but no other manifestations of sarcoidosis. How can I make a diagnosis?

## Question 45
We have read in your book that continuous oxygen therapy at home reduces mortality in chronic obstructive pulmonary disease (COPD). I am concerned that my patient might develop acute respiratory failure.

## Question 46
I have a patient with asthma who is on long-term inhaled corticosteroids. She is very concerned about long-term steroid therapy. Could I replace the steroids with a long-acting beta$_2$ agonist?

## Question 47
What is the role of leukotriene-modifying agents in asthma?

## Question 48
Is it true that the Mantoux test is no longer used?

## Question 49
Is there a screening test that is useful for the diagnosis of lung cancer?

## Question 50
For how long should treatment be continued for cervical lymphadenopathy and abdominal tuberculosis? What role, if any, do steroids play in the treatment of these conditions?

## Question 51
What is the recommended treatment for pleural mesothelioma?

## Question 52
- Why is there an increase in vocal fremitus and vocal resonance in consolidation?
- How are consolidation and pneumonia defined and are they the same thing?

## ANSWERS

### Answer 1
Alpha$_1$-antitrypsin inhibits neutrophil elastase, a proteolytic enzyme capable of destroying alveolar wall connective tissue. Alpha$_1$-antitrypsin deficiency allows damage to occur to distal lung tissue with the development of emphysema. Neutrophil elastase is the most abundant antiprotease in the lung and as smoking stimulates elastase release, lung tissue damage occurs leading to worsening emphysema.

### Answer 2
In bronchial breathing, the expiratory sound of breathing is louder on auscultation. In bronchiectasis due to collapse, dilatation and sometimes consolidation, the sounds are transmitted more directly through to the chest wall with little lung tissue to filter out the higher frequencies which are also characteristic of bronchial breathing.

### Answer 3
Consolidation allows the transmission of higher frequencies, which makes sounds like 'ninety-nine' clearer and often louder. Different countries have words of similar frequency to demonstrate this.

A pleural effusion decreases transmission of all breath sounds of whatever frequency and therefore little or no sound is heard.

### Answer 4
National Institute of Health and Clinical Excellence (NICE) UK guidelines state that nicotine replacement therapy or bupropion should only be used for the smoker who 'commits' to a stop date. Advice and encouragement to stop smoking should be offered. Both treatments are effective aids to stopping smoking; there is no evidence for their combined use. How bupriopion actually works here is unclear.

### Answer 5
Colds clear up within 1 week; rhinitis persists, being either seasonal or perennial.

Influenza is different from a cold. With a real episode of influenza the systemic effects of a temperature and muscle aches usually confine the patient to bed.

### Answer 6
Des-loratidine and levo-cetirizine are not available in the UK. Loratidine and cetirizine themselves are not teratogenic but loratidine is excreted in breast milk. To be on the safe side, no drugs should be used in pregnancy if possible.

## Answer 7

Acute bronchitis is literally inflammation of the bronchi; it is usually viral in origin. Pneumonia is inflammation of the lung substance and is most commonly due to bacteria; over 50% being due to *Streptococcus pneumoniae*.

## Answer 8

1. No, in such a sick patient steroid therapy should be continued, otherwise he or she will develop acute adrenal insufficiency, assuming that the patient has been on steroids for a long time.
2. No, there are no adverse reactions precluding the concurrent use of steroids.

## Answer 9

In COPD there is a reduction in the forced vital capacity (FVC) with a relatively greater reduction in forced expiratory volume ($FEV_1$).

## Answer 10

No; an obstructive pattern always reduces FVC.

## Answer 11

Clubbing does not occur in COPD. In a patient with COPD and clubbing, one would wonder whether a carcinoma of the bronchus, or bronchiectasis for example, were also present.

## Answer 12

Examination of the patient is helpful. Tachycardia, raised venous pressure, third and fourth heart sounds and basal crackles indicate cardiac failure. Chest wheezes suggest bronchospasm, and cough with sputum is more often seen in COPD. Exercise tests are helpful, as is the measurement of serum brain natriuretic peptide (BNP). A normal plasma level of BNP excludes heart failure. Response to therapy is often the best guide.

## Answer 13

There is a small element of bronchospasm, but the effect is small.

## Answer 14

There is no good reason for this but patients are very often anxious and this is the probable reason for them clawing their hands.

## Answer 15

No regimen of steroid usage is the best. Alternate-day administration has not been successful in asthma because patients can deteriorate during the

**Table 14.1** The stepwise management of asthma

| Step | Peak expiratory flow rate | Treatment |
|---|---|---|
| 1. Occasional symptoms, less frequent than once a day | 100% predicted | As-required bronchodilators If used more than once daily, move to step 2 |
| 2. Daily symptoms | ≤ 80% predicted | Anti-inflammatory drugs: Sodium cromoglicate or low-dose inhaled corticosteroids up to 800 µg If not controlled, move to step 3 |
| 3. Severe symptoms | 50–80% predicted | High-dose inhaled corticosteroids up to 2000 µg daily |
| 4. Severe symptoms uncontrolled with high-dose inhaled corticosteroids | 50–80% predicted | Add regular long-acting beta$_2$ agonist (e.g. salmeterol) |
| 5. Severe symptoms deteriorating | ≤ 50% predicted | Add prednisolone 40 mg daily |
| 6. Severe symptoms deteriorating in spite of prednisolone | ≤ 30% predicted | Hospital admission |

Short-acting bronchodilator treatment can be taken at any step on an as-required basis.

second 24 hours. There is certainly no need to give therapeutic steroids more than once daily except when initiating steroids for acute severe asthma. As with all drugs, it is best to get to know how to use the drug by seeing many patients. The stepwise management of asthma is shown in Table 14.1.

## Answer 16
Asthma must be well controlled during pregnancy and drugs should be given by inhalation to minimize exposure to the fetus. All drugs appear safe by inhalation. In acute attacks, parenteral steroids are safe and you should always keep the mother's oxygen saturation above 95% to prevent fetal hypoxia.

## Answer 17
Paracetamol.

## Answer 18
No.

## Answer 19
There are a number of different ways of classifying pneumonia. These include:
1. *Clinical*:
- Primary:
  - community acquired
  - hospital acquired.
- Secondary:
  - immunocompromised patients
  - aspiration pneumonia.
2. *Aetiological*: classified by infecting agent *(as in K&C 6e, Table 14.13, p. 923)*. The most common are: *Streptococcus pneumoniae* (50%), *Mycoplasma* spp. (6%), *Haemophilus influenzae* (5%).
3. *Anatomical*:
- Lobar.
- Segmental.
- Subsegmental.
- Bronchopneumonia.

## Answer 20
The classical description of typical pneumonia due to pneumococcus is:
- congestion
- red hepatization
- grey hepatization
- resolution.

The details of these are available in many books of pathology.

We dislike the term 'atypical' because it accounts for 20% of all pneumonias. The pathology in this group is not well described because very few patients die. The best description is by Parker et al. (1947).

*Reference*
Parker F, Jolliffe LS, Finland M (1947) Primary atypical pneumonia: report of 8 cases with autopsies. *Archives of Pathology* **44**: 581–608.

## Answer 21
It is unusual for the level of lymphocytes to drop below the normal range in aspiration pneumonia but obviously the total number of WBC and neutrophils do increase as a result of infection.

## Answer 22

No.

## Answer 23

SARS is due to a novel coronavirus, which is spread between humans by droplet infection. It is a zoonosis spread from small mammals, e.g. civet cats, raccoons. After initial non-specific symptoms, bronchopneumonia develops.

### Further reading

Guan Y et al. (2004) Molecular epidemiology of the novel coronavirus that causes severe acute respiratory syndrome. *Lancet* **363**: 99–104.

Ten separate articles on SARS appear in the *New England Journal of Medicine* **349** (2003).

## Answer 24

No symptoms will confirm the diagnosis of tuberculosis. A firm diagnosis can only be made by finding the tubercle bacillus in a specimen taken from the patient. Other features are only suggestive.

## Answer 25

Following infection with *Mycobacterium tuberculosis* the patient will develop cellular immunity to the organism. An intradermal injection of purified protein derivative (PPD) of *Mycobacterium tuberculosis*, usually in the forearm, will produce induration and inflammation at the site of the infection in such a patient. This reaction persists despite successful treatment of the disease. The reaction may not occur if the patient is very ill or develops AIDS, when the immune system is impaired.

## Answer 26

Following intradermal tuberculin challenge in a sensitized individual, antigen-specific memory T cells are activated to secrete interferon gamma (IFN-γ), which activates macrophages to produce more cytokines. BCG induces cellular immunity to the TB bacillus, which is an intracellular organism, in an *unsensitized* individual (Box 14.1).

## Answer 27

Sweats do mainly occur at night but patients often have a fever during the daytime but sweating is not prominent. Remember the commonest cause of night sweats is anxiety not an infective cause.

## Answer 28

Aspiration under ultrasound guidance should be performed, although 1 year's treatment is usually adequate.

---

**Box 14.1** **Tuberculin testing**

Mainly used for:
- Contact tracing
- BCG vaccination programmes

It is rarely of any value in the diagnosis of tuberculosis. Patients are tested with purified protein derivative (PPD) of *Myocobacterium tuberculosis*. The test is based on cell-mediated immunity with the development of induration and inflammation at the site of infection due to infiltration with mainly T lymphocytes. The test can be falsely negative in patients with AIDS because of impairment of delayed hypersensitivity.

**The Mantoux test**
- 0.1 mL of a 1 : 1000 strength PPD (equivalent to 10 tuberculin units) is injected intradermally.
- The induration (not the erythema) is measured after 72 hours. The test is positive if the induration is 10 mm or more in diameter.

**Whole blood interferon-gamma assay**
Can be used in all circumstances:
- In-vitro T cell basal assay
- T cells of individuals who have previously been sensitized to TB antigens will produce IFN-gamma when they are incubated with TB antigens (e.g. PPD)
- ELISA test or an enzyme-linked monospot assay
- Advantages:
  - no return visit to look at test
  - variable sensitivity and specificity

---

## Answer 29

Steroids are usually not recommended in these situations as there is insufficient evidence to know about their efficacy (Cochrane review).

## Answer 30

It is suggested that steroids might be beneficial here.

## Answer 31

Rifampicin should be stopped if the serum transferases, that is, the SGPT or alanine transferase (ALT) are raised more than three times normal. This is a rare situation.

## Answer 32

Fever should settle within 2 weeks. The ESR is usually normal within the month.

## Answer 33

The use of steroids is still controversial. In TB pericarditis, the European Society of Cardiology gives it a class II b recommendation (usefulness of efficacy less well established by evidence). The American Thoracic Society recommends steroids in the first 11 weeks. There is a growing base of clinical data for the use of steroids in meningitis; in one study it improved mortality.

## Answer 34

It is always tempting to use steroids in the conditions mentioned but the evidence is not convincing. They are said to reduce inflammation and tissue damage in pericarditis and meningitis (see above) but it is not currently recommended in pericarditis. For TB of the retina, systemic steroids are usually added to the ATT. Remember, you must not do harm with the use of drugs.

## Answer 35

Prednisolone dosage is variable. Prednisolone 30 mg daily often combined with azathioprine is a common regimen. Some clinicians use high doses, e.g. 1 mg/kg daily for 8–12 weeks but there is no good evidence that steroid therapy with or without azathioprine is beneficial. Methotrexate has also been used in place of azathioprine. A trial of both interferon-beta and interferon-gamma showed no benefit. Drugs that are being used include Bosentan (endothelin receptor antagonist), etanercept (a tumour necrosis factor-$\alpha$ receptor blocker) and imatinib [a platelet-derived growth factor (PDGF) inhibitor].

*Further reading*
Dempsey OJ et al. (2006) Idiopathic pulmonary fibrosis: an update. *Quarterly Journal of Medicine* **99**: 643–654.

## Answer 36

Concomitant connective tissue disorder usually with renal complications.

## Answer 37

Yes. Any disease that produces airflow limitation produces some wheeze on auscultation.

## Answer 38

No. The so-called 'barrel-shaped' chest is usually associated with kyphosis and old age rather than emphysema.

## Answer 39

Crocidolite fibres are long and thin and easily impact in the small airways where they are engulfed by macrophages. How exactly they get into the pleura is unclear, but they do because they can be found in pathological specimens.

## Answer 40
A pleural effusion produces stony dullness on percussion with reduced tactile vocal fremitus and vocal resonance over a wide area. Occasionally, it can be difficult and then ultrasound is helpful.

## Answer 41
A transudate is a fluid with protein content less than 30 g/L; an exudate has greater than 30 g/L. Other ways of expressing this are pleural fluid protein:serum protein ratio > 0.5 in exudates; a pleural fluid lactate dehydrogenase (LDH) > 200; or pleural fluid:serum LDH of > 0.6.

## Answer 42
In Meigs' syndrome, there is indeed some confusion. In Crofton and Douglas's *Respiratory Disease*, it is described as a transudate. It is likely that the pleural effusion has been formed by tracking of fluid through the diaphragm into the pleural space.

*Reference*
Meigs JV (1954) Fibroma of the ovary with ascites and hydrothorax; Meigs' syndrome. *American Journal of Obstetrics and Gynecology* **67**: 962.

## Answer 43
A major problem in cystic fibrosis is sputum infection with Burkholderia cepacia, a plant pathogen which was previously thought to be a harmless commensal. It's acquisition, however, can be associated with accelerated disease and rapid death. Sadly, this means that CF sufferers should not intermingle.

*Further reading*
Rowe S.M. et al. (2005) Mechanisms of disease: cystic fibrosis. *New England Journal of Medicine* **252**: 1992–2001.

## Answer 44
We assume you have done a serum angiotensin-converting enzyme level, which is elevated (75% of cases) of sarcoidosis. If this is not elevated, then biopsy confirmation is required. In your patient's case, this will be an endobronchial biopsy.

## Answer 45
You imply that your patient has hypercapnia. If this is the case you will have to give the oxygen via a 28% ventimask. If this is tolerated and blood gases show no rise in $PCO_2$, then you can increase the amount of inspiratory $O_2$ via a 34% mask.

## Answer 46

No! Fatalities have occurred in this situation. It would be reasonable to *add* a long-acting beta$_2$-agonist so that the inhaled steroids can be reduced. Patients should be warned about the possible exacerbation of their asthma that can occur with the addition of long-term beta$_2$-agonists.

## Answer 47

The clear indication for leukotriene modifying agents is in asthma due to aspirin sensitivity as these drugs inhibit lip oxygenase. A 2-week trial of one of these agents can be used to assess their effect on asthma control. If there is no improvement, the drug should be stopped.

## Answer 48

No. Tuberculin skin tests are still used but there is sometimes difficulty in interpreting the results. Whole-blood interferon gamma assays are being used. Their advantage is that they eliminate the error in interpreting the skin tests and only require a single visit.

## Answer 49

Yes, a recent study has shown that repeated annual spiral computerized tomography (CT) in smokers can detect lung cancer that is curable.

*Further reading*
Unger M (2006) A pause, progress and reassessment in lung cancer screening. *New England Journal of Medicine* **355**: 1763.

## Answer 50

For 6–9 months for extrapulmonary tuberculosis in a patient with organisms sensitive to the first-line drugs. Steroids have no part to play.

## Answer 51

Treatment of mesothelioma does not usually effect the median survival time of 6–12 months after presentation. Surgery (pleurectomy/decortication) and even more radical surgery with pre-and postoperative radiation and chemotherapy have all been tried without great success, good palliative care is essential.

## Answer 52

In consolidation, the lung is 'solid'. A solid lung conducts high-frequency sound better than air, which tends to dampen the high-frequency sound. As a result, vocal fremitus and vocal resonance are increased in consolidation with bronchial breathing being heard, which is a high-frequency sound. Pneumonia is defined as an inflammation of the substance of the lungs. The pathological process that occurs in the lungs as a result of the infection is called consolidation.

# Intensive care medicine 15

## QUESTIONS

### Question 1
Is there any role for heparin in management of septic shock?

### Question 2
Is there more adrenaline (epinephrine) or noradrenaline (norepinephrine) produced in shock? From where do these substances come from?

### Question 3
I hear conflicting views as to whether activated protein C is useful in shock.

### Question 4
Why does both vasoconstriction and vasodilatation occur in shock?

### Question 5
Are pulmonary artery (PA) catheters dangerous?

### Question 6
In most hospitals, what is the difference between a high-dependency unit (HDU) and an intensive care unit (ITU) and what is 'step down' care?

### Question 7
What is the difference between acute lung injury (ALI) and acute respiratory distress syndrome (ARDS) from a practical point of view?

### Question 8
What is the role of inhaled nitric oxide (NO) in acute respiratory distress syndrome (ARDS)?

## Question 9
What is meant by 'positive' pressure ventilation?

## Question 10
Why is an electroencephalogram (EEG) not used in all countries to evaluate possible brain death.

## ANSWERS

### Answer 1
There is no evidence of any effect on survival in any of the trials for the use of heparin in septic shock, and therefore it is not recommended.

### Answer 2
More adrenaline than noradrenaline is produced. Initially, this is from increased sympathetic nervous activity but this is later augmented by production of catecholamines from the adrenal medulla.

### Answer 3
You are correct, views are conflicting. Administration of recombinant human activated protein C was shown to improve survival in patients with sepsis-induced shock. A more recent study showed no benefit and the view now is that it should be tried if all else fails.

### Answer 4
The initial response in most forms of shock is release of catecholamines, which cause vasoconstriction, increased myocardial contractility and a tachycardia. There is later release of many vasoactive substances, e.g. nitric oxide, which causes vasodilatation.

### Answer 5
No; not when used by experts. There is, however, some evidence that PA catheters do not improve outcome and because of the complications and cost; it has been suggested that pulmonary artery catheterization has been overused.

### Answer 6
ITU means 'intensive' care with facilities to deal with multi-organ failure. The ratio between staff and patients is 1:1. In most hospitals, the ITU is also where invasive ventilation is performed if necessary. HDUs are often used postoperatively or when constant monitoring is required. They are sometimes used as a 'step down' from ITU before the patient is transferred to a ward.

### Answer 7
In ALI the $PaO_2/F_IO_2$ ratio is $<40$ kPA ($<300$ mmHg); in ARDS the ratio is $<26$ kPa ($<200$ mmHg). From a practical point of view, both are treated in the same way; respiratory support and treatment of the underlying condition.

### Answer 8
Inhaled nitric oxide reduces pulmonary artery pressure and improves V/Q mismatch. However it has not been shown to improve outcome.

*Further reading*
Rubenfeld GD et al. (2005) Incidence and outcomes of acute lung injury. *New England Journal of Medicine* **353**: 1685–1693.

## Answer 9

Gas is delivered under positive pressure into the airways during inspiration. It contrasts with negative pressure ventilation where the chest or whole body is encased in a tank to produce a negative airway pressure in inspiration.

## Answer 10

An EEG looks only at cortical activity, and loss of brainstem reflexes is necessary to confirm brain death. In the UK (but not the US) it is considered that an experienced clinician's examination of the patient makes an EEG unnecessary.

# Drug therapy and poisoning 16

**Question 1**
How should the body surface area be calculated when giving drugs for which doses are given per square metre of body surface area?

**Question 2**
Where can I find a reference table that shows drugs that can safely be prescribed and avoided during pregnancy and during lactation? Might this be included in the next edition of Kumar and Clark's *Clinical Medicine*?

**Question 3**
Where might I find a reference table showing paediatric drug doses?

**Question 4**
My question is concerned with the practical use of steroids. In inflammatory bowel disease, what doses are used and when is the dose reduced?

**Question 5**
What is the safe dosage/length of treatment for the drug dexmethasone so that its destructive effects are avoided?

**Question 6**
1. Please explain 'odds ratio' and 'risk ratio'.
2. What is meant by saying that diabetics have a 3.3 risk ratio of developing dementia?

**Question 7**
I'm a medical student from the Faculty of Medicine, Peradeniya, Sri Lanka. I have a question about the management of aspirin poisoning. Is it reasonable to carry out a postalkaline diuresis in these patients?

## Question 8
What is meant by intermediate syndrome in organophosphorus poisoning?

## Question 9
What are the pulmonary manifestations of Pink's disease and how common are they relative to the usual cerebral, skin and renal effects?

## Question 10
Is it necessary to administer antivenom to a person bitten by a snake 6 hours previously, presenting only with local leg swelling over the bitten site and so far no other systemic feature of poisoning?

## Question 11
What is the ideal management for scorpion bite?

## Question 12
In acute anaphylaxis, you recommend IM adrenaline (epinephrine). Surely in such an acute situation intravenous adrenaline would be better?

## Question 13
Why should patients avoid grapefruit juice if they are taking terfenadine?

## Question 14
Many older drug therapies, e.g. penicillin in streptococcal sore throat, have never been submitted to rigorous trials such as a randomized controlled trial (RCT). Do you think they should be?

## Question 15
Please explain why some drugs are teratogenic in the first trimester and some in the second?

## Question 16
What is the difference between compliance and concordance?

## Question 17
The rates of paracetamol (acetaminophen) self-poisoning have decreased in the UK. Why is this?

## Question 18
Is N-acetylcysteine of any use in a case of paracetamol overdosage taken 16 hours previously?

## Question 19
What is meant by primary end point and secondary end point?

## Question 20
Can chronic exposure to organophosphorus compounds (in farmers) cause axonal radiculoneuropathy persisting for years? Is this disease reversible?

## ANSWERS

### Answer 1
Body surface area is mainly used in children. The body surface area of a 70-kg man is $1.8\,m^2$. To calculate the dose in a child use the following formula:

$$(\text{Surface area of patient } (m^2) \times \text{adult dose}) \, 1.8$$

However, the best way to ensure the correct dose in children is to use reference tables or the manufacturer's guidelines.

### Answer 2
In the UK, the *British National Formulary* (BNF) contains the data you ask for, as does the reference book *Martindale: the Complete Drug Reference*, edited by Sean C Sweetman. The information can also be found in Kumar and Clark's *Handbook of Medical Therapeutics*.

### Answer 3
In the UK, this information can be found in the *British National Formulary* (BNF) and in the reference book *Martindale: the Complete Drug Reference*. In addition, it is also available in paediatric textbooks and manufacturers' information sheets.

### Answer 4
There are no hard and clinically proven rules for the use of steroids (usually prednisolone) in inflammatory bowel disease; there is also no fixed way to reduce the dose. In moderate/severe inflammatory bowel disease we start with 45 mg prednisolone as a single dose daily for 1 week, reducing this to 30 mg daily for 2 weeks and then by 5-mg decrements, depending on the clinical condition of the patient and the changes in inflammatory markers, e.g. erythrocyte sedimentation rate and C-reactive protein.

### Answer 5
There is no safe dosage/length of treatment, particularly with a potent steroid like dexmethasone. For example, ischaemic necrosis of bone has been described after three doses of dexmethasone 4 mg. You must always keep the dose as low as possible for as short a time as possible.

### Answer 6
1. The odds ratio (OR) is the ratio of the probability of an event occurring to the probability of an event not occurring. The probability itself is an estimate of the likelihood of an event, usually expressed as a number between 0 and 1.

Thus, when calculating the OR, it is the odds of, for example, an adverse event occurring in the treated group, i.e. the number with an adverse event (a) divided by the number without the event (b), divided by the odds of the event occurring in the placebo group, i.e. the number of controls with adverse events (c), divided by the number without (d). Thus:

$$OR = (a/b) \div (c/d)$$

The risk ratio (RR) is the 'rate' of the event occurring in the treated group, i.e. the number on treatment with, for example, a drug getting an adverse reaction (a) divided by the total number (a + number with no reactions) (b). This is divided by the rate of the event occurring in the control group on a placebo – again, the number on placebo getting an adverse event (c) – divided by the total number on treatment (c and d (number with no reaction). Thus, the RR or relative risk is:

$$a/(a \text{ and } b) \div c/(c \text{ and } d)$$

(See *K&C 6e, p. 1000* for an explanation of odds ratio.) In the same example, the risk ratio would be [a/(a + b)] ÷ [c/(c + d)].
2. A risk ratio of 3.3 means a 3.3 increased risk of developing dementia in this case.

## Answer 7
Plasma salicylate levels should be performed in all patients suspected of aspirin overdosage.
   Plasma salicylate levels of 500–700 mg/L (3.62–5.07 mmol/L) at 2 hours, 4 hours (or later) after aspirin ingestion should have urine alkalinization (*see K&C 6e, p. 1009*) with 225 mL of an 8.4% bicarbonate infused over 1 hour. Forced alkaline diuresis should no longer be used.

## Answer 8
The intermediate syndrome consists of cranial nerve and brainstem lesions with a proximal neuropathy, which starts 1–4 days after acute intoxication and lasts 2–3 weeks. Respiratory failure due to muscle weakness can occur. The aetiology is uncertain but is probably due to inadequate treatment.

## Answer 9
Pink's disease is due to mercury ingestion in the old teething powders and therefore infants were affected. You will need to check with a paediatric specialist. The disease does not now occur in many countries because the compounds are no longer available.

## Answer 10
Antivenoms are not usually required unless signs of systemic env`enoming are present. There are, however, exceptions to this rule and

rapid progression of swelling is one. If systemic signs are present it is never too late to give antivenom. You must get expert local advice.

## Answer 11
Pain from the sting can be helped by local anaesthetic (local infiltration or ring block). Parenteral analgesia is also required frequently. The use of antivenom is controversial.

## Answer 12
Adrenaline has a rapid onset of action. It is well absorbed from the IM route, even in shocked patients. For these reasons it is a much safer option than IV adrenaline, which can be dangerous.

## Answer 13
Grapefruit juice inhibits the P450 enzyme CYP3A4. This is due to the interaction between flavinoids and other chemicals that are found in grapefruit. Interaction between the antihistamine terfenadine means that the two should never be given together. However, this is academic because terfenadine has been withdrawn because of its cardiac effects.

## Answer 14
Let us not forget that many patients' lives have been saved by antibiotics such as penicillin. Good observational studies are still relevant. It would, of course, be extremely difficult to do an RCT now in many situations, e.g. penicillin for a streptococcal throat infection.

## Answer 15
Teratogenicity only occurs in the first trimester (particularly 3rd–11th weeks), causing congenital malformation. Following this, drugs can affect growth and functional development of the fetus but this is not teratogenic.

## Answer 16
Compliance simply means that patients are not taking the drug prescribed. Concordance is a more general term implying an implicit agreement between the doctor and the patient on the value of taking therapy.

## Answer 17
There are many reasons; one being the education about the dangers of the drug. In addition, you cannot buy more than 16 tablets at any one time from drug outlets in the UK. Foil-wrapped drugs are also less likely to be taken for self-harm.

### Answer 18
Yes there is evidence that continued infusion of N-acetylcysteine improves the morbidity and mortality of liver problems, even after 16 hours (Fig. 16.1 and Box 16.1).

### Answer 19
The main result is measured at the end of the study to see if the treatment has worked, e.g. mortality in the treatment group versus the placebo group. This primary end point should be clear before the study starts. The secondary end point refers to other variables, such as side-effects in the treatment group, which might affect the overall results.

### Answer 20
There has been much debate about the effects of chronic exposure to organophosphate compounds. Chronic low exposure might cause neurological lesions, but these changes are subtle. Acute exposure does cause axonal damage to roots and peripheral nerves.

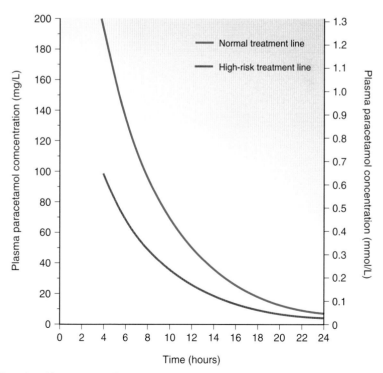

Fig. 16.1 Nomogram of paracetamol. From *British National Formulary* (1998) with permission.

---

**Box 16.1** Antidote regimens for paracetamol poisoning

**_N_-acetylcysteine (intravenously in 5% glucose)**

- 150 mg/kg in 200 mL over 15 min, then 50 mg/kg in 500 mL over the next 4 hours and 100 mg/kg in 1000 mL of 5% glucose over the ensuing 16 hours
- Total dose: 300 mg/kg over 20.15 hours

_Note_: A 48-hour regimen is used in some US centres: patients receive a loading dose of 140 mg/kg, followed by 70 mg/kg every 4 hours for 12 doses, all infused over 1 hour

**_N_-acetylcysteine (orally)**

- 140 mg/kg initially, then 60 mg/kg every 4 hours for 17 additional doses
- Total dose: 1300 mg/kg over 72 hours

**Methionine**

- Oral 2.5 g followed by three similar doses every 4 hours if unable to give _N_-acetylcysteine

---

# Environmental medicine 17

**Question 1**
In view of the controversial reports on the use of melatonin for long distance flights, I would like to know if the editors use it?

**Question 2**
What are Osborn waves?

**Question 3**
Why does there appear to be a high incidence of cancer of the thyroid gland but not other areas following the Chernobyl nuclear accident in 1986?

**Question 4**
I read that death is more likely in a drowning accident in fresh rather than sea water. Is this true?

**Question 5**
Is it dangerous to use MP3 players?

## ANSWERS

### Answer 1
We do travel a lot and have therefore read the studies on melatonin with great interest. We have not tried it ourselves mainly because of the conflicting data. Friends who have used it say the timing of the dose is crucial.

### Answer 2
These are the J waves (hypothermic waves) that are seen on the electrocardiogram in hypothermia. They are rounded waves that occur immediately after the QRS complex and are pathognomonic of hypothermia.

### Answer 3
Large doses of radioactive iodine appear to have been released; iodine is concentrated in the thyroid gland.

### Answer 4
No. Although originally it was thought that there were differences related to the hypertonicity of sea water pulling fluid into the lungs, it is now thought that the severe hypoxaemia is related to the amount of water aspirated.

### Answer 5
This depends on loudness and the duration of use. It is suggested that 80 decibels is the upper limit for possible damage. MP3 players can reach 105 decibels, although there is a sound limiter on European models. It is suggested that you should take a break after 1 hour of listening. Remember, hearing damage will not become evident for months or years.

## QUESTIONS

### Question 1
Is growth hormone deficiency in childhood commonly associated with panhypopituitarism?

### Question 2
I would like to ask why, when treating hypopituitarism, an adrenal crisis occurs if thyroid replacement is given before steroid replacement therapy? And what is the underlying mechanism? Thank you!

### Question 3
Why, in Sheehan's syndrome, is there an anterior pituitary involvement more than a posterior one?

### Question 4
Is the cyclic presence of Montgomery tubercles, where they reduce and later increase, in a nulliparous woman's breast normal? And, if so, what is the cause?

### Question 5
Does methyltestosterone, if given in a daily dose of 2.5 mg per day, cause liver cell injury or hypothalamic gonadal suppression? Can this drug be prescribed for other cases with hypothalamic hypogonadism, usually being given by intramuscular injection or implant?

### Question 6
Does IM testosterone increase levels of serum thyroid-stimulating hormone (TSH)?

### Question 7
For some time now I have been confused regarding tests for acromegaly.

1. Which is best – screening or diagnosing test in these patients?
2. Your book says the 'glucose tolerance test [GTT] is diagnostic'. Does this mean GTT with growth hormone (GH) evaluation or that a patient who is clinically an acromegalic with a positive GTT (diabetic) can be labelled as acromegalic?

Incidentally, a lot of people around me are similarly confused and others have been following the latter saying that 'Kumar and Clark say so'. Please clarify.

## Question 8
Does acromegaly cause depression?

## Question 9
1. Breathlessness can be a feature of acromegaly. What are the characteristics of this breathlessness?
2. If a patient presents with headaches due to acromegaly, what are the likely characteristics of these headaches?

## Question 10
Why does hypothyroidism cause a transudative pleural effusion?

## Question 11
What is the significance of the thyroid-releasing horomone (TRH) test in differentiating various causes of hypothyroidism?

## Question 12
Is retention of urine/incomplete voiding related to hypothyroidism? If so, how?

## Question 13
It is stated that a little overtreatment might be required for hypothyroidism, i.e. slightly raised thyroxine (T4) and suppressed thyroid-stimulating hormone (TSH). Is the clinical improvement the best criteria or is there an optimum/maximum level that one should watch out for when monitoring TSH and T4?

## Question 14
Why is thyroid-stimulating hormone (TSH) normal or increased in patients with peripheral resistance to tri-iodothyronine (T3) and thyroxine (T4)? The thyroid hormone levels are high in these patients, so the TSH should drop lower: why doesn't it?

## Question 15
Thyroxine is a peptide hormone used to treat thyroid deficiency and other thyroid disorders. It is taken orally. Peptides are broken down into amino

acids before being absorbed. What factors cause the thyroxine to remain stable in the digestive tract so that it is absorbed without being digested?

## Question 16
1. Does the absence of bradycardia exclude hypothyroidism?
2. How often is hypothyroidism accompanied by bradycardia?

## Question 17
Should patients with hypo- or hyperthyroidism be given iodine supplements?

## Question 18
Is Hashimoto's thyroiditis associated with dementia?

## Question 19
Please explain the causes of, and suggest recommended treatments for, euthyroid and hypothyroid states.

## Question 20
What is the role of propranolol in the management of a 35-year-old male thyrotoxic patient who is also hypertensive?

## Question 21
What else could we use instead of propranolol in thyrotoxicosis with bronchial asthma?

## Question 22
At what dose, and for how long, would steroid therapy give rise to secondary adrenal insufficiency? For adrenal insufficiency due to long-term steroid use, when should we start to give a cortisone supplement? How should we monitor these patients?

## Question 23
What dose of Synacthen is equivalent to adrenocorticotrophic hormone (ACTH)?

## Question 24
I want to know the mechanism that causes anaemia in Addison's disease. I am unable to find the real cause.

## Question 25
What causes hypercalcaemia in Addison's disease?

## Question 26
In the diagnosis of Cushing's disease using the high-dose dexametha-sone suppression test, how can the exogenous steroid suppress

adrenocorticotrophic hormone (ACTH) when the grossly elevated serum cortisol levels fail to do so?

## Question 27
Does alternate-day therapy with steroids decrease their efficacy compared with daily therapy?

## Question 28
Regarding the renin–angiotensin–aldosterone axis, it states that dietary sodium excess suppresses renin secretion. Then why are we asking hypertensives to restrict sodium intake? Also if we are using angiotensin-converting enzyme (ACE) inhibitors, the plasma renin activity increases due to loss of feedback inhibition. Wouldn't that be counterproductive?

## Question 29
How does a phaeochromocytoma give rise to Raynaud's phenomenon?

## Question 30
How well do symptoms of hypercalcaemia correlate with serum calcium levels. Can I ignore an asymptomatic patient with a serum calcium of 3.7 mmol/L but have to give treatment to a symptomatic patient who has a serum calcium of 3.3 mmol/L?

## Question 31
A 64-year-old woman tells me she has been on hormone replacement therapy (HRT) – oestrogen only following a hysterectomy – for 7 years. She wants to continue with this therapy as she thinks it helps her. How long should I continue prescriptions?

## Question 32
Is there a difference between impotence and erectile dysfunction and are the treatments different if they are different conditions?

## Question 33
In multiple endocrine neoplasia under screening, you say that family members who are 'at risk' should be screened. What does that mean?

## Question 34
You mention that a number of tests can be used in the diagnosis of a phaechromocytoma. Can you say which is the best and do they all need to be done, considering the expense of those investigations?

## Question 35
In a patient who is found to be hypertensive, how should we exclude Conn's syndrome?

## Question 36

Diabetes mellitus and diabetes insipidus are very different conditions so why are they both called diabetes?

## Question 37

I have a young patient who has hirsutism associated with the polycystic ovary syndrome. She has become desperate about her symptoms, which have not been improved by long-term medical treatment with oestrogens, spironolactone and cyproterone. She has asked about whether surgery would help.

## Question 38

In a previously fertile patient with infertility secondary to testosterone replacement, how soon after stopping testosterone therapy will he become fertile again? Can reduced fertility and hypogonadism be treated other than with testosterone replacement therapy?

## Question 39

Why is the 'insulin-like growth factor' (released from the liver in response to the growth hormone) so called, although it opposes the effects of insulin?

## Question 40

Does hyperprolactinaemia cause gynaecomastia?

## ANSWERS

### Answer 1
Growth hormone deficiency in children is usually an isolated defect but pituitary deficiency can occur and should be treated.

### Answer 2
Thyroid replacement therapy increases cortisol degradation and basal metabolism. This can precipitate an adrenal crisis if steroids are not given first.

### Answer 3
Sheehan's syndrome is now very rare. There is anterior pituitary involvement rather than posterior because the blood supply to the anterior pituitary is dominant.

### Answer 4
Yes, it is normal. Montgomery's tubercles respond to oestrogens. Hyperpigmentation or overdevelopment are other signs of hyperoestrogenism.

### Answer 5
This is a small dose; liver damage is unlikely. Pituitary gonadotrophin secretion inhibition does occur. Testosterone is used in hypothalamic hypogonadism.

### Answer 6
Intramuscular testosterone does not affect serum TSH.

### Answer 7
1. An undetectable growth hormone level excludes acromegaly. The best diagnostic test is either an oral GTT with measurement of growth hormone levels or a single raised plasma insulin-like growth factor 1 (IGF-1) level.
2. In patients with diabetes mellitus (who therefore have a diabetic GTT) *without* acromegaly the IGF-1 levels are low, whereas in a diabetics *with* acromegaly the IGF-1 levels are high. Kumar and Clark is correct.

### Answer 8
No; prolonged symptoms can 'depress' people, as in any other illness, which can be difficult to diagnose.

### Answer 9
1. The breathlessness is usually due to cardiac disease, which is a feature of acromegaly.

2. The headaches are due to pituitary tumours. The headaches are variable. They can be felt behind the eyes or on top of the head.

## Answer 10
In hypothyroidism there is generalized water retention and this can produce a pleural effusion that is a transudate.

## Answer 11
The TRH test was used to differentiate thyroid from hypothalamic/pituitary causes of hypothyroidism. It has been replaced by accurate measurement of serum thyroid-stimulating hormone, making the TRH test obsolete.

## Answer 12
No; retention of urine is not a feature of hypothyroidism.

## Answer 13
Clinical improvement is certainly of value but this should be backed up with TSH and T4 estimations. These should be kept within the normal range. A TSH above 10 mmol/L usually requires an increase in T4. Most patients with hypothyroidism require 150 μg of T4 daily.

## Answer 14
There seems to be resistance at the pituitary gland as well, so feedback is reduced.

## Answer 15
Thyroxine is a small peptide that is absorbed intact, as are many other small peptides. Although some proteins are broken down into peptides and then individual amino acids, many small peptides are absorbed intact.

## Answer 16
1. No.
2. Severe hypothyroidism is often associated with bradycardia (60%) but many cases are now diagnosed on the evidence of high levels of thyroid-stimulating hormone and low serum thyroxine, with few clinical signs.

## Answer 17
Iodine would be appropriate where dietary deficiency of iodine still exists. Iodine in the form of potassium iodide (60 mg three times daily) is given prior to thyroidectomy for hyperthyroidism but there is little evidence for its beneficial effect!

## Answer 18
Rarely; usually there is mental slowness. All dementia patients must be screened for hypothyroidism with a serum thyroid-stimulating hormone.

## Answer 19
Euthyroid means normal thyroid function and requires no treatment! Hypothyroid is usually due to an autoimmune cause and low/decreased thyroid function. Thyroxine is used for replacement therapy.

## Answer 20
It means you can treat both conditions with one drug. Instead of discontinuing propranolol when the patient is euthyroid, continue it to control blood pressure.

## Answer 21
Propranolol should not be used in bronchial asthma, as you indicate. A cardioselective beta-blocker such as atenolol or metoprolol can be used with extreme caution. Remember, beta-blockers are mainly given for symptom control until the definitive therapy (e.g. antithyroid drugs, radioactive iodine) has controlled the hyperthyroidism. Thus, some patients do not need beta-blocker therapy.

## Answer 22
There is no definite figure for how long steroid therapy needs to be given before secondary adrenal insufficiency occurs. However, it is very unlikely on less than 3 weeks of treatment. You only need to give steroid cover for severe illness or for surgery (*see K&C 6e, p. 1084*). A stimulation test with adrenocorticotrophic hormone is not normally required.

## Answer 23
1 mg tetracosactide (Synacthen) is equivalent to 80 units of ACTH in terms of adrenal stimulation.

## Answer 24
The normocytic, normochromic anaemia that occurs in patients with Addison's disease is probably a direct effect of glucocorticoid deficiency. In addition, as most cases are due to autoimmune disease, the anaemia can be due to pernicious anaemia.

*Further reading*
Burke CW (1985) Adrenocortical insufficiency. *Clinics in Endocrinology and Metabolism* **14**: 947–976.

## Answer 25
Many factors, including increased bone resorption and increased calcium resorption by proximal tubules, both of which are partly mediated by

glucocorticoids. Mild to moderate hypercalcaemia occurs in 6% of patients and is corrected by glucocorticoid replacement therapy which increases renal excretion.

*Further reading*
Muls E et al. (1982) Etiology of hypercalcemia in a patient with Addison's diseases. *Calcified Tissue International* **34**: 523–526.

## Answer 26
The 'grossly' elevated cortisol level is still in the nanomolar level. Oral dexamethasone is given as 1 mg.

## Answer 27
No; alternate-day therapy is used to try to reduce the side-effects of steroids. Do not use in asthma.

## Answer 28
Dietary sodium reduction will raise renin levels, although not invariably. Increased blood pressure (BP) levels have been observed in some hypertensive patients when dietary sodium is reduced. This heterogeneity in BP response has led some authorities to divide patients into 'salt sensitive' or 'salt resistant'. Elderly patients who might have low renin levels often show reduction in BP on sodium restriction. The action of ACE inhibitors in preventing the formation of angiotensin II is more important than the renin effect.

## Answer 29
High circulating levels of noradrenaline (norepinephrine) produce vasoconstriction.

## Answer 30
Patients with hyperparathyroidism are often asymptomatic. There is, therefore, no good correlation between symptoms and serum calcium levels. In patients with acute hypercalcaemia, often due to malignancy, symptoms usually develop rapidly. You should therefore treat any patient with acute hypercalcaemia with symptoms or any patient with a serum calcium of greater than 3.5 mmol/L (normal range is 2.20–2.67 mmol/L or 8.5–10.5 mg/dL).

## Answer 31
This is often an individual decision, which must be made jointly between you and the patient. You should inform the patient of the risks, which are:
- Breast cancer risk increased by 1.5 extra cases per 1000 over 5 years (normal risk is 14 per 1000).

- Venous thrombosis risk increased by 4 extra cases in 1000 cases (normal risk 20 per 1000) over 5 years.
- Stroke incidence rises by 6 extra in 1000 (normal risk number 20 cases).

The patient must balance these risks against any perceived benefits.

*Further reading*
Grady D (2006) Management of menopausal symptoms. *New England Journal of Medicine* **355**: 2338–2347.

## Answer 32
The term 'impotence' includes both loss of libido and erectile dysfunction. A lack of libido is a loss of sexual desire leading to erectile dysfunction. The treatment for erectile dysfunction is now a phosphodiesterase type 5 inhibitor, e.g. sildenafil, which can also help with the loss of libido. Additional measures might be required for loss of libido.

## Answer 33
The family members 'at risk' are those who have the gene mutation.

## Answer 34
The first and most useful screening test is the measurement of urinary catecholamines and metanephrines in two 24-hour urine collections. Normal levels virtually exclude the diagnosis. (*Note*: many drugs and dietary vanilla interfere with the test.) Following a positive test, imaging, i.e. computed tomography or magnetic resonance imaging, should be performed.

## Answer 35
60% of patients with Conn's syndrome have hypokalaemia along with their hypertension. These patients, along with all hypertensives under 35 years, require investigation. The best screening test is the plasma aldosterone : renin ratio, which is elevated.

## Answer 36
Diabetes is derived from a Greek word meaning a siphon. It means excessive urination 'like the passing of water by a siphon', which occurs with both conditions.

## Answer 37
Wedge resections of ovaries were used in the past with very poor results. Metformin has improved hirsutism in some patients. Presumably she has already tried local therapies.

*Further reading*
Rosenfield RL (2005) Hirsutism. *New England Journal of Medicine* **353**: 2578–2588.

## Answer 38

Yes; spermatogenesis recurs in weeks after the drug is stopped; whether the patient becomes fertile again depends on many factors. Luteinizing hormone, follicle-stimulating hormone and pulsatile gonadotrophin-releasing hormone are all used when fertility is required (*see K&C 6e, p. 1055*).

## Answer 39

Insulin-like growth factor (IGF) is a polypeptide about the same size as insulin. IGF-1, IGF-II and insulin genes are part of the same family. IGF-I, IGF-II and human proinsulin have some structural similarities, which explain their different activities.

## Answer 40

Yes. Gynaecomastia can occur in men with hyperprolactinaemia; rarely galactorrhoea.

# 19 Diabetes mellitus and other disorders of metabolism

## QUESTIONS

### Question 1
I would like to know the exact mechanism of entry of potassium into cells under the influence of insulin.

### Question 2
I am seeing an increasing number of diabetic patients in primary care who have elevated fasting blood glucose readings but postprandial measurements that are normal or only slightly high. Does this indicate insulin resistance in these patients? What is the reason for this trend?

### Question 3
What are the latest diagnostic criteria for the diagnosis of diabetes mellitus?

### Question 4
What test is recommended for diabetes and can the same be used to diagnose diabetes in a child?

### Question 5
What is the value of glycosylated haemoglobin ($HbA_{1C}$) in diabetes mellitus?

### Question 6
I read in a book that in diabetics the random blood sugar is more important than the fasting; on a medical website I noted that, for a patient with type 2 diabetes, the fasting blood sugar level is more important. What do you say?

Is it acceptable to let the fasting blood sugar remain at approximately 1.5 mmol/L above the upper limit in a patient of $> 60$ years with type 2 and presently on oral therapy?

## Question 7

In type 2 diabetes, which blood sugar – fasting or random – is more revealing prognostically?

## Question 8

Why are the fasting and 2-hour blood glucose levels needed in a diabetic patient being treated with oral antidiabetic drugs?

## Question 9

Is it sufficient to use a fasting blood sugar and glycosylated haemoglobin (HbA$_{1C}$) level as a guide to modify the insulin or oral antidiabetic dose without considering the 1 and 2 hour postprandial values?

## Question 10

What is the value of the 2-hour postprandial blood sugar level above which the dose of an oral antidiabetic should be increased if this value is exceeded several times despite dietary modification?

## Question 11

What does BM mean in relation to blood sugar monitoring?

## Question 12

What is the role of urine examination in diabetic control?

## Question 13

Diabetes and diet: could the authors of my favourite medical text please advise whether or not it is acceptable to have controlled quantities of refined sugar, providing the total calorie intake is kept under control?

## Question 14

Do non-obese patients with impaired fasting glucose, i.e. a glucose level of 6.1–6.9 mmol/L, need drug treatment with biguanides if lifestyle modifications fail to normalize?

## Question 15

Do non-obese patients with impaired glucose tolerance (but not fulfilling the criteria for diabetes mellitus) need drug treatment with biguanides if lifestyle modifications fail to normalize their post-prandial blood glucose measurements?

## Question 16

It is the Muslim month of fasting currently. I would be grateful if you could advise on how to adjust the insulin regimen of a type 1 diabetic patient, for example a 21-year-old girl who is on subcutaneous Actrapid (short-acting soluble insulin) 22 units t.d.s.

## Question 17

I would like to know more about the use of the glitazone group in type 2 diabetes: its action, side-effects, precautions taken on using them.

## Question 18

In a patient receiving oral antidiabetics, should the drug be administered just after taking the blood sample for fasting blood glucose level (and before a meal), or just prior to the sample being taken?

## Question 19

What oral antidiabetics are safe in pregnancy?

## Question 20

Is it necessary to put all type 2 diabetics on aspirin?

## Question 21

In the chapter on diabetes you wrote that you should avoid tablets before age of 40 years in non-insulin-dependent diabetes mellitus (NIDDM). Why is this, because in our country most doctors are prescribing this?

## Question 22

1. Should a patient poorly controlled on glibenclamide 15 mg a day and metformin 1500 mg a day be moved onto insulin?
2. What are the indications for insulin in type 2 diabetics?

## Question 23

What happens to the insulin-secreting capacity of a type 2 diabetic placed on insulin therapy earlier than recommended? Can the external supply of insulin improve the functional capacity of the insulin-secreting cells, to some extent by providing some rest to these cells?

## Question 24

1. Is inhaled insulin a suitable substitute for injectable insulin?
2. Is there, or will there soon be, insulin in the form of a tablet?

## Question 25

What are the complications of insulin other than hypoglycaemia and injection?

## Question 26

I would like to know the processes that go into administering the Alberti's/modified Alberti's regime in patients with uncontrolled diabetes mellitus.

## Question 27

Is there any role for steroids in the management of resistant diabetes mellitus (daily insulin requirement exceeding 100 units/day)? Don't they make glycaemic control worse?

## Question 28

What is the importance of potassium chloride (KCl) in the treatment of a diabetic patient (pre-operative care)? The formula in the text is explained as 16 U of insulin + 10 mmol of KCl + 500 mL 10% glucose.

## Question 29

What is the cut-off point of daily albumin excretion above which a diabetic patient without hypertension should be given an angiotensin-converting enzyme (ACE) inhibitor?

## Question 30

What is the urinary concentration or 24-hour urine albumin content above which angiotensin-converting enzyme (ACE) inhibitors should be started in diabetic patients? Does an albumin (in microgram)/creatinine (in milligrams) ratio above 30 in the morning sample indicate a need for this?

## Question 31

Do potassium channel activators such as nicorandil have any benefit in the treatment of a diabetic patient with cardiovascular complications?

## Question 32

Is a dosage of 2.5 mg/day of methyltestosterone, as a component in some multivitamin formulae, safe to give to diabetics or will it make the diabetes more difficult to control (see also Chapter 5, question 5)?

## Question 33

How does diabetes mellitus cause atherosclerosis?

## Question 34

How does diabetes cause renal damage, especially diabetic nephropathy with the presence of microalbuminuria?

## Question 35

Type 1 diabetes causes nephropathy in 40% of cases and type 2 causes it in 20% of cases but the most common cause of nephropathy we see is type 2, why?

## Question 36

Why is intractable vomiting seen in diabetes mellitus and how can it be managed?

## Question 37
Is gabapentin superior to carbamazepine in terms of efficacy in the treatment of painful diabetic neuropathy? What are its side-effects?

## Question 38
Why is diabetic ketoacidosis more common in type 1 diabetes?

## Question 39
Why is there abdominal pain in diabetic ketoacidosis?

## Question 40
Grades of ketonuria are sometimes mentioned. I have not been able to locate a detailed description in textbooks and would be grateful if you could explain the grades of ketonuria or recommend suitable reading material.

## Question 41
What false-positive factors could cause ketone bodies to appear in the urine in a non-diabetic patient?

## Question 42
Why is tetanus not seen in a diabetic foot wound?

## Question 43
Can impaired glucose tolerance cause recurrent lower motor facial palsy?

## Question 44
Can long-term diabetes mellitus cause vertigo not accompanied by other brainstem signs?

## Question 45
We know that type 2 diabetes mellitus provokes left ventricular diastolic dysfunction. Does chronic stable angina, associated with type 2 diabetes mellitus, further increase the prevalence of left ventricular diastolic dysfunction?

## Question 46
Is there adequate evidence for choosing an angiotensin-converting enzyme (ACE) inhibitor or antagonist for the initial management of raised blood pressure in type 2 diabetes, or is it now advisable to choose any tolerated antihypertensive?

## Question 47
Why is there immunosuppression in diabetes?

## Question 48
Dextrose infusion in quinine induced hypoglycaemia causes more hypoglycaemia, so what is to be used?

## Question 49
Does the serum cholesterol level rise with age?

## Question 50
Please explain the significance of having normal total high-density lipoprotein (HDL) and low-density lipoprotein (LDL) cholesterol but a raised lipoprotein (a) [Lp(a)] in a normotensive, non-smoking patient?

## Question 51
In the diet of hypercholesterolaemic patients, should milk and other dairy products be restricted?

## Question 52
Should a 20-year-old, either male or female, with a blood cholesterol level of 300 mg/dL and with hypercholesterolaemic parents, be treated?

## Question 53
Why are lipid-lowering drugs (statins) administered at bed time?

## Question 54
What is the best statin now and what is your opinion about Crestor 10 mg (rosuvastatin) and Lescol XL (fluvastatin sodium)?

## Question 55
How long do statins take to achieve their maximum benefit?

## Question 56
If, after 4 months of taking simvastatin (20 mg daily), a patient with hyperlipidaemia and hypertension has an increased aspartate transferase (AST) of up to 60 U/L, with a normal alanine transferase (ALT), what action should I take?

## Question 57
How long should the statins be continued once the lipid profile returns to normal? Can we stop the statins once normal levels are attained and then continue with diet modification?

## Question 58
What is the exact mechanism of corneal arcus? What is its clinical significance? What is its relationship to hyperlipidaemia? Is there any

effective treatment in medicine or alternative medicine to remove
corneal arcus?

### Question 59

What is the best drug to be added to a statin in a case of familial
hypercholesterolaemia not responding to lifestyle and diet modification
plus a statin?

### Question 60

Can diabetes mellitus cause Horner's syndrome? If so, how?

### Question 61

Is it typical for a diabetic patient to experience angina during myocardial
ischaemia?

### Question 62

What are the causes of a flat oral glucose tolerance test (GTT)?

### Question 63

Are there any indications for routinely prescribing a statin (simvastatin,
for example) in hypertensive and/or diabetic patients as prophylactic
therapy?

### Question 64

What are the causes of vomiting and other gastrointestinal tract problems
in type 2 diabetes mellitus? What is the correct treatment for a patient
with nausea and vomiting, already taking hypoglycaemic agents and
antihypertensives?

## ANSWERS

**Answer 1**
Insulin promotes active transport of glucose into the cell (using the glucose transporter GLUT 4) and this is accompanied by potassium transport.

**Answer 2**
We can see no reason for the change that is occurring in your primary care practice. The difference between fasting and postprandial measurements might be related to insulin resistance in type 2 diabetes but it also relates to changes in lifestyle, i.e. food intake and exercise.

**Answer 3**
The diagnosis for diabetes mellitus is a fasting plasma glucose greater than 7 mmol/L (126 mg/dL) or random plasma glucose greater than 11.1 mmol/L (200 mg/dL). The two abnormal values that are required in an asymptomatic patient to indicate impaired glucose tolerance are shown in Box 19.1.

**Answer 4**
The diagnosis is made on:-symptoms of diabetes and a random plasma glucose of >200 mg/dL (11.1 mmol/L or a fasting plasma glucose >126 mg/dL (7.0 mmol/L). This also applies to children.

**Answer 5**
Glycosylation of haemoglobin results in the formation of a covalent bond between the glucose molecule and the terminal valine of the beta chains of the haemoglobin molecule. The rate at which this occurs is related to the prevailing glucose concentration. $HbA_{1C}$ is expressed as a percentage of the normal haemoglobin, and normal is 4–8%. This test provides an index of the average blood glucose concentration over the life of the haemoglobin molecule, about 6 weeks. It therefore gives a more general picture of the blood glucose level than a single blood glucose.

---

**Box 19.1** Definitions

**Impaired fasting glucose (IFG)**
American Diabetes Association criteria is a plasma glucose level of
5.6–6.9 mmol/L (110–126 mg/dL)

**Impaired glucose tolerance (IGT)**
Fasting plasma glucose <7 mmol/L (126 mg/dL) at 2 h. At 2 h following a 75-g glucose load: 7.8–11 mmol/L (140–200 mg/dL)
*Note*: both IFG and IGT are risk factors for the development of diabetes and cardiovascular disease

## Answer 6

Both the random blood sugar and the fasting blood sugar are of some use in the management of type 2 diabetes. However, both are isolated measurements. It is much more useful to get patients to measure their own blood glucose three or four times a day, say at 3-weekly intervals. An alternative is to use the glycosylated haemoglobin level, which is the best guide to overall blood sugar levels over the preceding 3 months. In both type 1 and type 2 diabetes, good control reduces the risk of complications. Your patient should therefore be encouraged to keep a normal blood sugar and a normal level of glycosylated haemoglobin.

## Answer 7

Any high blood sugar, whether fasting or random, indicates diabetes but single tests, e.g. in the clinic, are of limited value. Help your patients to do their own blood testing at home.

## Answer 8

It is better to use the glycosylated haemoglobin ($HbA_{1C}$) level; the ideal is <7% and the patient does not need to be fasted.

## Answer 9

The best approach is for the patient to do blood sugars at home throughout the day, with $HbA_{1C}$ being performed at the clinic visit.

## Answer 10

Two-hour postprandial blood sugar is not as good a measurement as $HbA_{1C}$, which should be less that 7%. If the level is higher, the oral diabetic therapy should be increased if possible. However, do not hesitate to start insulin therapy sooner rather than later.

## Answer 11

BM stands for Boehringer Mannheim, the firm that produces a number of glucose measurement strips.

## Answer 12

Glycosuria occurs when the blood glucose level exceeds the renal threshold. This threshold varies, and fluid intake affects urine glucose concentration. A negative urine does not distinguish between hypo-, normo- or even slight hyperglycaemia. For these reasons, diabetic control is monitored using blood samples obtained at regular intervals by the patient. However, in a stable type 2 diabetic whose urine is always negative and occasional blood glucose tests are normal, urine tests can be used if the patient refuses to do regular blood tests.

## Answer 13
No, it is not a good idea because refined sugar will produce abrupt swings in glucose level due to rapid absorption. Better to eat an apple!

## Answer 14
Impaired fasting glucose carries the same risks of cardiovascular disease and future onset of diabetes as impaired glucose tolerance. So, yes, metformin is used in these patients.

## Answer 15
Impaired glucose tolerance is a risk factor for future diabetes and cardiovascular disease. Therefore, many diabetologists start metformin therapy (Fig. 19.1).

## Answer 16
Fortunately, the Muslim faith does not require insulin-dependent diabetic patients to fast during Ramadan. Some patients do, however, decide they would like to fast.

One regimen is for the patient to run on a bed-time injection of insulin glargine. This long-acting insulin acts over approximately 24 hours and will often provide sufficient basal insulin to carry the patient through from bed time to the evening of the next day. The size of the insulin glargine (basal) injection is adjusted during the year to get pre-breakfast blood glucose readings of 5–7 mmol/L.

On top of the basal insulin, the patient injects a rapid-acting, rapidly disappearing insulin whenever he or she eats. During the year this will be three times a day. During Ramadan it will be twice a day (before sunrise and after sunset).

The meal-time insulin is adjusted to the size of the meal on the plate, aiming to get a home blood glucose reading of 5–8 mmol/L 2 hours postprandially. Trial and error is needed for each patient to be able to 'guestimate' how much insulin goes with a meal of a given size. This regimen is also used in shift workers.

## Answer 17
Pioglitazone and rosiglitazone are the two glitazones available in the UK. They act by reducing peripheral insulin resistance. The current recommendations are that glitazones should be used in patients who are unable to take metformin and a sulphonylurea, or for those whose blood sugar remains high on this combination.

There are rare reports of liver dysfunction, and monitoring of liver biochemistry is necessary every 2 months for the first year. These drugs can also cause salt and water retention, giving oedema and rosiglitazone has been linked with increased cardiac events.

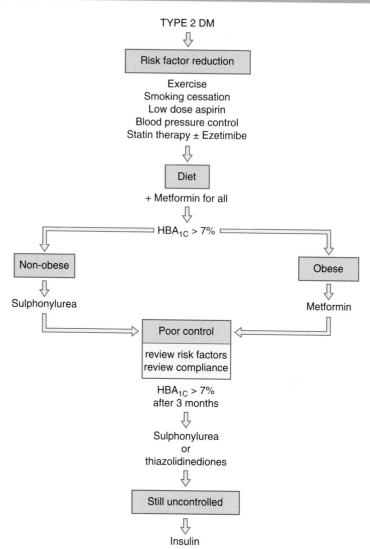

Fig. 19.1 A treatment pathway for type 2 diabetes mellitus.

**Answer 18**

It makes no difference.

**Answer 19**

Glibenclamide was shown in one trial to be safe in pregnancy; it does not cross the human placenta. However, most diabetologists do not use oral therapy in pregnancy.

## Answer 20

No, it is not always necessary. However, the group of patients over 50 years of age with a coronary heart disease risk greater than 15 over the next 10 years will include many people who are diabetics, and they should be given low-dose aspirin.

## Answer 21

The statement that you should 'avoid tablets before the age of 40 years' is a reference to the fact that below 40 years most patients have type 1 diabetes with insulin deficiency and therefore require insulin therapy.

## Answer 22

1. Yes – use insulin in all type 2 patients if glycosylated haemoglobin ($HbA_{1C}$) is >9.0%. It is better to start insulin therapy early than to wait.
2. Failure of control using oral agents, including the glitazones. Weight gain is a problem with insulin therapy.

*Further reading*
Nathan DM (2006) Thiazolidinediones for initial treatment of type 2 diabetes? *New England Journal of Medicine* **355**: 2477–2480.

## Answer 23

Beta-cell function steadily decreases in type 2 diabetes. No improvement in functional capacity of beta-cells would occur with insulin therapy.

## Answer 24

1. Inhaled short-acting insulin is being used by some but it is not in general use. Its use is probably as an adjunct and it is unlikely that injection therapy will be totally avoided.
2. Insulin, like other proteins, is broken down in the gut so oral insulin is not feasible unless some special coating of the tablet could be found. Nothing is in sight at the moment.

## Answer 25

There are very few complications. Antibodies can be demonstrated in the serum but rarely cause a problem. Patients can react to the protamine added to make long-acting insulins. Weight gain can be a problem and needs to be monitored because many patients feel hungry.

## Answer 26

In 1976, Alberti published a paper on using small doses of either intramuscular or intravenous insulin for the treatment of diabetic ketoacidosis. Prior to this, large doses of insulin had traditionally been used.

## Answer 27
There is no role for steroids, even in resistant diabetes.

## Answer 28
Insulin therapy drives $K^+$ into the cell and hypokalaemia can result. Hence always give $K^+$ 20 mmol/L of 0.9% saline.

## Answer 29
30–300 mg in 24 hours is called microalbuminuria. In type 1 diabetes, if microalbuminuria is persistent despite good glycaemic and lipid control, an ACE inhibitor should be used. In type 2 diabetes, an ACE receptor blocker is preferred.

## Answer 30
Frank proteinuria, i.e. >300 mg/day, should be treated with an ACE inhibitor/antagonist after good glycaemic and lipid control has been instituted. A ratio of 30 would also indicate the necessity for treatment.

## Answer 31
Nicorandil probably is no better than any of the other drugs that are used for the treatment of angina.

## Answer 32
2.5 mg methyltestosterone is a very small dose and should be safe in diabetics. It is, however, difficult to see an indication for this therapy.

## Answer 33
The mechanism of atherosclerosis is not clear but probably includes:
- Endothelial dysfunction.
- Abnormalities of coagulation, particularly in the fibrinolytic pathway.
- Plaque composition: there is increased lipid and macrophages in plaques in diabetes mellitus which increase the risk of rupture.
- Platelet activation leading to aggregation.

*Further reading*
Gaede P et al. (2003) Multifactorial intervention and cardiovascular disease in patients with type 2 diabetes. *New England Journal of Medicine* **348**: 383–393.

## Answer 34
The pathogenesis of the renal complications of diabetes mellitus is still not completely understood.

In general, the conversion of glucose to sorbitol via the polyol pathway seems to play a central role as this leads to vascular permeability and structural defects in capillaries.

In the kidney, the glomerular filtration rate (GFR) is initially increased out of proportion to plasma flow owing to an elevation in the transglomerular pressure gradient. The raised glomerular pressure might promote transglomerular passage of proteins as well as glycosylate end products. This could lead to proliferation of mesangial cells and accumulation of matrix products in the basement membrane. These are the first changes seen pathologically when microalbuminuria occurs. These changes eventually lead to glomerular sclerosis with progressive loss of glomeruli and more marked proteinuria.

## Answer 35

You are correct, but there are of course many more cases of type 2 diabetes; hence this is the most common cause.

## Answer 36

Delayed gastric emptying has been demonstrated in approximately 50% of unselected usually asymptomatic patients with type 1 diabetes. There is usually evidence of an autonomic neuropathy and often a peripheral neuropathy. There is, however, no good correlation between the motility findings and the symptoms. A few patients do develop severe vomiting. In addition, hyperglycaemia *per se* inhibits gut motility.

Treatment consists of very good glycaemic control. Metoclopramide, domperidone or erythromycin (this acts on motilin receptors) can also be tried. Hospital admission is occasionally required for dehydration and control of diabetes.

## Answer 37

Gabapentin is effective in painful neuropathy, although trials are small. It produces many side-effects (look up your national formulary) but on the whole is well tolerated. It does cause troublesome diarrhoea. Carbamazepine is also effective but less so. Only two drugs have been approved by the US Food and Drug Administration based on phase III RCTs: pregabalin (related to gabapentin) and duloxetine, which inhibit the receptors of serotonin and noradrenaline (norepinephrine).

## Answer 38

In type 1 diabetes there is no or very low insulin available. In type 2, insulin is present although there is resistance to its action. This is the reason for diabetic ketoacidosis in type 1 diabetes.

## Answer 39

The cause of abdominal pain in diabetic ketoacidosis is not clear.

## Answer 40

In ketoacidosis, stix testing of the urine will show very high ketone levels (grade III). This is occasionally useful if you have any doubt of the diagnosis. Low levels of ketonuria (grade I) are seen in starvation.

You can also measure ketone levels in the serum; again high ketone levels are seen in ketoacidosis.

## Answer 41
Starvation is the main cause. It also occurs after heavy alcohol consumption (starvation is also involved as people do not eat when drinking heavily).

## Answer 42
The diabetic foot ulcer is not usually caused by trauma where the tetanus bacillus can be picked up. It is usually the result of neuropathy and/or ischaemia.

## Answer 43
There is some evidence that neuropathies can occur without overt diabetes mellitus.

## Answer 44
It depends on the cause of the vertigo. If the vertigo is due to a brainstem vascular lesion associated with diabetes mellitus, nystagmus is frequently present. Transient vertigo occurs with hypoglycaemia without the neurological signs.

## Answer 45
Type 2 diabetes is associated with coronary artery disease, which usually produces left ventricular systolic dysfunction with some degree of diastolic dysfunction. In chronic stable angina, the diastolic dysfunction is usually stable except after exercise when 'demand ischaemia' occurs due to increased oxygen demand when there is a decreased coronary flow.

## Answer 46
There is good evidence that ACE inhibitors or angiotensin receptor antagonists are renoprotective. Recent guidelines suggest that the antagonists should be used first in type 2 diabetes.

## Answer 47
Type 1 diabetes is an immune mediated disease and there is some immunosupression. It has been shown that treatment with an immunosuppressive drug prolongs beta cell survival, although this is not used in clinical practice.

## Answer 48
Quinine overdose can cause hypoglycaemia but dextrose (10%) infusion can be used and will prevent severe hypoglycaemia in most cases. The mechanism of the hypoglycaemia is increased insulin secretion. Intramuscular glucagon might be of short-term help and Octreotide 50 μg SC 6-hourly has been used.

## Answer 49
Yes.

## Answer 50
LP(a) is associated with an increased risk of coronary heart disease, but in the patient you describe, who has a normal cholesterol, nothing should be done.

## Answer 51
Milk and other dairy products should be restricted. However, it is only with severe restriction that a significant effect on cholesterol levels is seen and this is often unacceptable to patients. Some restriction, plus a statin, may be a better option.

## Answer 52
Yes, with diet and a statin (Table 19.1).

## Answer 53
Cholesterol synthesis is maximal in the late evening/early morning, so that giving a statin at night maximizes its effect.

## Answer 54
There is no best statin. When prescribing drugs it is usually wise to use the drug you know best, not to go immediately for the newest.

## Answer 55
At least 4 weeks.

## Answer 56
None; treatment should only be discontinued if transferases are more than three times the upper limit of normal.

**Table 19.1** Target goals of risk factors for diabetic patients (standards from the American Diabetes Association, 2003)

| Parameter | Ideal | Reasonable but not ideal |
|---|---|---|
| HbA$_{1C}$ | <7% | <8.5% |
| Blood pressure (mmHg) | <130/80 | <140/90 |
| Total cholesterol (mmol/L) | <4.5 | <6 |
| LDL | <2.6 | |
| HDL* | >1.1 | |
| Triglycerides | <1.7 | <2.0 |

* In women, >1.3 mmol/L.
HbA$_{1C}$, glycosylated haemoglobin; HDL, high-density lipoprotein; LDL, low-density lipoprotein.

### Answer 57
Probably forever, as diet modification seldom works.

### Answer 58
Lipid/cholesterol deposits in the cornea produce an arcus. In the young, it is said to be associated with hyperlipidaemia but the exact relationship is unclear. It has no significance in the elderly as it is a degenerative process. There is no treatment.

### Answer 59
A number of patients with familial hypercholesterolaemia do need an additional drug. Ezetimibe (a cholesterol absorption inhibitor) should be added to a statin.

### Answer 60
No. Diabetic neuropathy is described on p. 1128 of Kumar and Clark *Clinical Medicine* 6th edn, and the sympathetic nervous system can be involved in diabetes. However, Horner's syndrome is not described.

### Answer 61
Diabetic patients classically have 'silent' ischaemia or heart attacks due to the accompanying neuropathy. They can, however, have typical angina with chest pain.

### Answer 62
A flat oral GTT occurs when there is malabsorption of glucose. It was used in the 1950s and 1960s as a test to show malabsorption. However, it was replaced by tests using non-metabolized sugars, such as xylose, which were more reliable. More recently, absorption tests have been superseded by imaging, antibody tests and histology of the small intestine to diagnose malabsorptive conditions such as coeliac disease.

### Answer 63
Most patients with hypertension and diabetes will require a statin but before starting this agent you should encourage lifestyle changes, e.g. stopping smoking, taking regular exercise and reducing fat in the diet. Use statins to keep serum cholesterol to $<4$ mmol/L (150 mg/dL).

### Answer 64
Vagal damage can lead to gastroparesis but this is usually in type 1 diabetes. There is no correct treatment for nausea and vomiting; meal changes and antiemetics are the best approaches.

# The special senses 20

## QUESTIONS

### Question 1
Does central vertigo decrease with time?

### Question 2
Are vestibular sedatives such as betahistine indicated in the treatment of benign paroxysmal positional vertigo?

### Question 3
Does the absence of nystagmus in Hallpike's manoeuvre exclude benign paroxysmal positional vertigo (BPPV), even in the presence of a typical clinical picture and an absence of other possibilities? Does wearing Frenzel's goggles increase sensitivity?

### Question 4
With Ménière's disease, what steps should be taken:
1. In acute attacks?
2. Before an attack starts?

### Question 5
I want to ask about the proven medicine for tinnitus in UK.

### Question 6
Why do patients with Goldenhar's syndrome experience speech delay, despite the fact that they might be able to use their unaffected ear to listen with?

### Question 7
In sinusitis, it is not the nasal cavity that is congested by excessive mucus but the openings between the paranasal sinuses and nasal cavity. Why, therefore, does sinusitis cause difficulty breathing?

## Question 8
What is the modern treatment and prognosis for glaucoma.

## Question 9
What is the recommended treatment for slow age-related macular degeneration of the eye?

## Question 10
What does the term pseudo-papilloedema mean?

## Question 11
Could direct ophthalmoscopy falsely detect papilloedema due to error of refraction?

## Question 12
What is the cause of bilateral macular oedema?

## Question 13
How can one differentiate between papilloedema and a tilted disc on fundus examination?

## Question 14
On fundus examination, does the preservation of the disc cup (no obliteration) despite nasal blurring of the edges of the cup mean an absence of papilloedema?

## Question 15
What findings should be looked for during routine fundus examination in patients on long-term chloroquine or other anti-malarial therapy for treatment of systemic lupus erythematosus (SLE)?

# ANSWERS

## Answer 1
Most patients with vertigo improve within days but continuous true vertigo with nystagmus suggests a central lesion. Physiotherapy helps the 'compensation' process by the brain.

## Answer 2
No; the best treatment is the Epley manoeuvre, which consists of gentle but specific manipulation and rotation of the patient's head to shift the loose otoliths from the semicircular canals.

## Answer 3
The absence of nystagmus would bring the diagnosis into doubt, although the sensitivity of the Hallpike manoeuvre is variable (50–80%). Frenzel's goggles are used to prevent visual fixation, which suppresses nystagmus due to a peripheral lesions such as BPPV; they might help.

## Answer 4
1. In an acute attack, give cinnarizine.
2. Low-salt diet, avoid caffeine, try betahistine.

## Answer 5
The treatment is that of the underlying cause, e.g. removal of earwax, treatment of otitis media. Drugs (e.g. betahistine dihydrochloride) are often used; their benefit is variable. Carbamazepine and phenytoin are used in persistent cases. Intolerable tinnitus can sometimes be masked by a hearing aid.

## Answer 6
Many have middle ear defects with impairment of hearing in addition to the change in the ear itself.

## Answer 7
There are two reasons: first, the sinusitis is usually secondary to an upper respiratory tract infection (often viral); second, there is nasal obstruction. Both of these will cause difficulty with breathing.

## Answer 8
Primary open-angle glaucoma is the common type and of course it does lead to irreversible blindness (Box 20.1). The aim of treatment is to reduce the intra-ocular pressure. This can be done either by reducing aqueous production (with a topical beta-blocker, e.g. timolol) or increasing aqueous drainage (uveoscleral outflow) with a prostaglandin analogue,

---

**Box 20.1 Loss of vision: summary**

**Painless loss of vision**
- Cataract
- Open-angle glaucoma
- Retinal detachment
- Central retinal vein occlusion
- Central retinal artery occlusion
- Diabetic retinopathy *(see K&C 6e, p. 1124)*
- Vitreous haemorrhage
- Posterior uveitis
- Age-related macular degeneration
- Optic nerve compression
- Cerebral vascular disease

**Painful loss of vision**
- Acute angle-closure glaucoma
- Giant cell arteritis *(see K&C 6e, p. 1249)*
- Optic neuritis *(see K&C 6e, p. 1181)*
- Uveitis
- Scleritis
- Keratitis
- Shingles
- Orbital cellulitis
- Trauma

---

latanoprost. Sympathomimetics and carbonic anhydrase inhibitors are also used. Reduction in the intraocular pressure reduces visual loss. Apart from medical treatment, laser therapy and surgery are used but without good evidence of their efficacy.

*Further reading*
Leske MC et al. (2003) Factors for glaucoma progression and the effect of treatment. *Archives of Ophthalmology* **121**: 48.

## Answer 9

A number of treatments have been introduced for neovascular (or wet) age-related macular degeneration (ARMD) in the last few years. Photodynamic therapy with verteporfin was the first to show a decrease in visual loss. This has, however, been superseded by bevacizumab and ranibizumab, both monoclonal antibodies that neutralize endothelial growth factor A. They are very expensive.

*Further reading*
Brown DM et al. (2006) Ranibizumab versus verteporfin for neovascular related macular degeneration. *New England Journal of Medicine* **355**: 1432–1444.

## Answer 10
The term is sometimes used for conditions that simulate disc oedema.

## Answer 11
Long-sighted refractive errors make the disc appear pink and ill-defined. Opaque (myelinated) nerve fibres at the disc margin and hyaline bodies can be mistaken for disc swelling.

*Further reading*
Wong T, Mitchell P (2007) The eye in hypertension. *Lancet* **369**: 425–435.

## Answer 12
Diabetes mellitus is the most common cause. There is gradual onset of blurring of vision. Fundoscopy often shows no other evidence of retinopathy. Annual visual acuity should be checked.

## Answer 13
Venous congestion is present in true papilloedema. Fluorescent retinal angiography is occasionally necessary to show true papilloedema.

## Answer 14
Preservation of disc cup – no papilloedema.

## Answer 15
The early changes are macular oedema, increased pigmentation and granularity of the retina. The characteristic lesion is a central area of depigmentation of the macula surrounded by an area of pigmentation – a 'bull's eye lesion'. This is usually accompanied by visual disturbances.

# 21 Neurological disease

## Question 1
Please what is (are) the likely cause(s) of sudden sharp but brief pain (resembling pin prick) in the right lower abdomen?

## Question 2
What are the causes of foot drop, and what is the likely treatment?

## Question 3
What is the correct definition for dysaesthesia?

## Question 4
What is the difference between 'light touch' and 'fine touch' sensations passed in the posterior column, and which one of these is tested with a wisp of cotton?

## Question 5
What is apraxia of gait and what is Brun's apraxia?

## Question 6
Why is it that, when eliciting the plantar reflex, we are supposed to stop just before the ball of the great toe?

## Question 7
Is there any rationale for giving dopamine agonists to aphasic patients?

## Question 8
Have either carbamazepine or dopamine agonists a role in the treatment of aphasia? If yes, what type of aphasia?

## Question 9
Is bilateral VIth cranial nerve palsy always a false-localizing sign (i.e. does it indicate an increased intracranial pressure and not pathology of the nerves or their nuclei)?

## Question 10
Can an optic tract lesion, which is mononuclear field loss (i.e. loss of vision in one eye) also be called 'incongruous homonymous hemianopia'?

## Question 11
How would you treat optic neuritis?

## Question 12
After two episodes of optic neuritis, one affecting each eye and 2 months apart, confirmed to be demyelinating in nature by visual evoked potentials, could a diagnosis of multiple sclerosis be reached in the absence of periventricular lesions on the MRI?

## Question 13
While assessing the pupillary reflexes, the consensual light reflex is really difficult to see in the other eye. Are there any tips for that?

## Question 14
Is it clinically significant to examine the consensual light reflex? If there is a lesion of the IIIrd cranial nerve of the unilluminated eye to impair the consensual response, this will be clear by the other symptoms and signs of the IIIrd cranial nerve palsy on that eye. If there is a lesion of the optic nerve of the unilluminated eye, the patient will not have a direct light reflex of that eye when examining its own direct reflex. I am not sure how the IIIrd cranial nerve can lose only its parasympathetic fibres. It is difficult to see the unilluminated pupil when light is not directly shining on it.

## Question 15
Should every patient with trigeminal neuralgia be given an MRI of the brain?

## Question 16
Is carbamazepine more effective than phenytoin in the treatment of trigeminal neuralgia? Would this patient need a higher dose of carbamazepine, and what is the upper limit?

## Question 17
Is gabapentin effective in the treatment of trigeminal neuralgia?

## Question 18

What medication is best used for the treatment of carbamazepine-resistant trigeminal neuralgia?

## Question 19

What are the common causes of recurrent lower motor facial nerve palsy?

## Question 20

In a case of facial nerve palsy, what is the value of preserved taste sensation? Does its preservation exclude upper motor affection and/or nuclear lesion or is it localized between the facial canal and the cerebellopontine angle?

## Question 21

Can Synacthen be used instead of steroids in the treatment of idiopathic Bell's palsy and how long should the treatment last? What is the recommended dose?

## Question 22

Is aciclovir a helpful treatment for idiopathic Bell's palsy?

## Question 23

In a child aged 5 years, can the presence of horizontal, fine, bilateral nystagmus with the fast component towards the point of fixation, with no other neurological or system abnormality, be considered a normal variant?

## Question 24

Are inner ear sedatives, and betahistine in particular, effective in the treatment of vertigo due to lateral medullary syndrome or any central lesion?

## Question 25

Are steroids appropriate in the treatment for vestibular neuronitis?

## Question 26

Why is there no gag reflex during the act of deglutition as I have seen that when we touch any thing to the posterior third of the tongue there is always gag reflex?

## Question 27

Can cerebellar lesions cause head nodding? Is this involuntary movement diagnostic for a cerebellar lesion in a patient who does not display Parkinsonian features or essential tremor?

## Question 28

1. What is the treatment of choice in symptomatic myoclonus resulting from a lesion of the cerebral cortex or spinal cord?
2. Does piracetam have a role in treatment of symptomatic myoclonus resulting from lesion of the cerebral cortex or spinal cord?

## Question 29

Is ankle clonus diagnostic of pyramidal tract lesion?

## Question 30

Is pronator drift pathognomonic of a pyramidal tract lesion or does it occur with any lesion of the motor system?

## Question 31

Can proximal muscle weakness be more than that of the distal muscles in cases of upper motor neurone lesions?

## Question 32

In the absence of either myopathy or radiculopathy, could a pyramidal tract lesion be diagnosed despite a distribution of weakness that is proximal more than distal?

## Question 33

Are brisk deep tendon reflexes, rather than hyperreflexia, pathognomonic of pyramidal tract lesion?

## Question 34

What is Wartenberg's reflex (sign), and is it diagnostic of a pyramidal tract lesion?

## Question 35

Must an extensor plantar response be present in order to diagnose a pyramidal tract lesion even in the presence of weakness of pyramidal distribution and other pathological reflexes?

## Question 36

Is it common to find Babinski's sign positive in Todd's paralysis?

## Question 37

In a case of paraplegia owing to an upper motor neuron lesion, does the ability of the patient to sit indicate intact thoracic segments?

## Question 38
Can the Brown–Séquard syndrome be diagnosed with pyramidal weakness of one lower limb and hypoaesthesia of the other lower limb but with no dissociative sensory loss of the hypoaesthetic limb?

## Question 39
Is there more than one method of demonstrating dysdiadochokinesia in upper limbs?

## Question 40
What is the difference between kinetic and intention tremors?

## Question 41
What is the best treatment for rubral tremors besides treating the aetiology?

## Question 42
What is meant by 'inversion of reflexes'? I have found this term in a few membership exams.

## Question 43
Is it possible for patients with posterior column lesions to be suffering from allodynia, with pain on pressure to different musculoskeletal points? Or is this more likely to be caused by fibromyalgia?

## Question 44
How do the clinical success rates of gabapentin and carbamazepine compare?

## Question 45
What clinical tests can be done to determine dissociative sensory loss?

## Question 46
What is the recommended dose of urograffin before performing contrast-enhanced computed tomography? How far in advance should this be administered before imaging when an intracerebral abscess or glial tumour is suspected?

## Question 47
How many urografin ampoules (76% concentration) should be administered before a CT brain scan with contrast searching for a mass lesion, and how many minutes before imaging should these be injected?

## Question 48
1. What is the difference between fluid-attenuated inversion recovery (FLAIR) and T2-weighted MRI scans?

2. What is the advantage of magnetization transfer pulse over a FLAIR MRI scan?

## Question 49
Does lumbosacral MRI refer to lumbosacral spines or to lumbosacral cord segments?

## Question 50
What type of painful stimuli can be applied in calculating the Glasgow Coma Scale for both motor and eye-opening responses, and how should these be applied?

## Question 51
How can the Glasgow Coma Scale be assessed in a patient with receptive or expressive aphasia?

## Question 52
How common is it for someone suffering a transient ischaemic attack (TIA) to totally lose consciousness? Also, what is the mechanism for losing consciousness with a TIA?

## Question 53
What should the management be for a stenosis in the carotid artery causing transient ischaemic attack (TIA), and when is surgery recommended?

## Question 54
In a patient with central retinal artery branch occlusion with carotid artery stenosis, what is the best management: warfarin, aspirin or carotid endarterectomy?

## Question 55
If a young patient who has suffered a stroke has a normal mental state, would this exclude a cerebral venous occlusion as an aetiology?

## Question 56
Does persistent hiccough following cerebrovascular ischaemic stroke localize to the medulla or to any other site?

## Question 57
By what mechanism is vertebrobasilar insufficiency associated with circumoral numbness?

## Question 58
Why does lateral medullary syndrome result in ipsilateral diplopia due to cranial nerve VI?

## Question 59

I have seen many established ischaemic stroke patients with CT-documented capsular infarction and hemi-hypotonia despite exaggerated reflexes. How would you explain the hypotonia? Could it be due to a corticorubral fibre lesion?

## Question 60

Thrombolytic therapy is used in patients with a cerebral infarct within the first 3 hours, whereas stroke by definition lasts > 24 hours. So how do we define that it is infarct and not a transient ischaemic attack (TIA) on a CT scan within the first 3 hours in order to start tissue plasminogen activator (tPA) treatment?

## Question 61

I want to ask something about cerebrovascular accident (CVA). Can you please tell me how we can rapidly pinpoint the exact anatomical site of the neurological deficit using physical findings in the emergency room?

## Question 62

Why do you treat dissection of the carotid artery with an anticoagulant in the acute management of stroke secondary to dissection? To me this seems paradoxical as it would increase the severity of dissection.

## Question 63

Last week, in a neurology viva, I was asked about the indications for heparinization in patients with a stroke. I want to know when I can stop heparin and what test I should use for assessing its therapeutic range.

## Question 64

Has heparin a role in the management of acute ischaemic stroke not accompanied by atrial fibrillation?

## Question 65

1. In the treatment of a stroke, does low-molecular-weight heparin (LMWH) have an advantage over heparin?
2. In an ischaemic stroke in evolution, for how long should heparin be administered?

## Question 66

Can streptokinase be used in acute cerebral infarction and, if so, what is the dose?

## Question 67

There seems now to be a consensus about starting aspirin therapy in acute ischaemic strokes as early as possible. Why has this changed from past recommendations to avoid aspirin early (during the first 48 hours) during the ischaemic stroke on the pretext that it could convert an ischaemic infarct into a haemorrhagic one, thus increasing the dangers of complications like cerebral oedema and raised intracranial pressure? If both opinions are based on clinical trials, what is the significance of the much hyped 'evidence-based medicine'?

## Question 68

I understand that a loading dose of clopidogrel 600–900 mg can be given to ischaemic stroke in evolution and can stop the evolving deficit. Would you agree?

## Question 69

Is there any rationale for giving patients with recurrent strokes a combination of aspirin and anticoagulant?

## Question 70

1. Does a dipyridamol–aspirin combination have any superiority over aspirin alone in the secondary prevention of a stroke?
2. Is an aspirin plus anticoagulant combination superior to a dipyridamol–aspirin combination in the treatment of recurrent ischaemic stroke not controlled by aspirin alone?

## Question 71

1. Is it safe to give piracetam to patients with primary intracerebral haemorrhage? Does it have a neuroprotective effect?
2. Is it safe to give a patient with excessively high blood pressure (as a sequela to recent primary intracerebral haemorrhage) angiotensin-converting enzyme inhibitors to lower the blood pressure?
3. Is it indicated to give piracetam or vincamine to a patient with middle cerebral artery territorial infarction? Do these have any neuroprotective effect?

## Question 72

What is the mechanism by which subarachnoid haemorrhage is associated with subhyaloid haemorrhages on fundus examination, and how can cerebrospinal fluid (CSF) gain access to the subhyaloid space inside the eye?

## Question 73

What is the recommended dosage for nimodipine given intravenously in cases of subarachnoid haemorrhage, and when should the treatment start? For how long should the dose be continued?

## Question 74

I read recently that hyperuricaemia has something to do with stroke? Is it recommended to give allopurinol to stroke patients irrespective of their serum uric acid?

## Question 75

Is there a link between hyperuricaemia (although asymptomatic) and atherosclerosis and cerebral ischaemic stroke?

## Question 76

Are phenytoin and carbamazepine indicated in myoclonus, occasionally seen in ischemic strokes?

## Question 77

What is the treatment of chorea or action myoclonus resulting from embolic stroke to the area of basal ganglia? Does the L-dopa that is given by some neurologists improve the condition? Does valproate have a role if the case is action myoclonus?

## Question 78

How should a patient with a haemorrhagic cerebrovascular accident be managed while also having an extensive inferior wall myocardial infarction?

## Question 79

What is the best way to manage cortical vein thrombosis? If heparin is to be used, what is the recommended dosage and how long should this treatment last?

## Question 80

In the case of cortical vein thrombosis, for how long should anticoagulation be continued?

## Question 81

How long should antiepileptic treatment be continued for a stroke patient who has the first seizure within the first 24 hours of the stroke?

## Question 82

For how long should antiepileptic drugs be given to patients having their first seizure within the first week of their cerebrovascular stroke?

## Question 83

What are the causes of epilepsy with a normal electroencephalogram (EEG), other than metabolic causes? Could epilepsy due to CNS causes be associated with a normal EEG? Could epilepsy due to the gradual withdrawal of an antiepileptic drug occur as much as 1 year later?

## Question 84
What are uncinate fits?

## Question 85
Are epileptic fits occurring strictly during sleep pathognomonic for frontal or temporal lobe epilepsy or any other epileptic syndrome?

## Question 86
Despite childhood somnambulism often disappearing later in life, could its first presentation after puberty on a nearly daily basis, raise the possibility of frontal lobe epilepsy or other organic pathology? Would an electroencephalogram (EEG) or polysomnography confirm this?

## Question 87
Could masticatory automatisms follow a generalized tonic–clonic fit? If so, would these or would these not be considered part of the same fit?

## Question 88
Is it common for epileptic patients to have postictal vomiting? If so, how often does this occur?

## Question 89
In temporal lobe epilepsy, what is meant by 'cephalic aura' and how does this manifest itself?

## Question 90
What is the difference between pseudoseizures and pseudo-pseudoseizures?

## Question 91
Does a delay in controlling seizures result in more frequent seizures and a more resistant epileptic disorder? And, if so, does this apply to all seizure types?

## Question 92
What genetic tests are recommended for epilepsy and Huntington's disease?

## Question 93
Is it useful to take an electroencephalograph (EEG) after a patient's first-ever seizure and, if so, when is the best time to do so? Would you recommend taking an EEG after every seizure and before diagnosis?

## Question 94
How often can drop attacks with loss of consciousness be due to atonic fits in the absence of any other type of fit?

## Question 95
How often are atonic fits the cause of falls with loss of consciousness in a patient not suffering from any other type of seizure?

## Question 96
Can mild anaemia (haemoglobin 10.8 g/dL) in a young female cause syncopal attacks that are preceded by a sense of falling, followed by a loss of consciousness and drowsiness for up to 1 hour? Do these data favour complex partial seizures rather than syncope?

## Question 97
I am confused between simple and complex partial seizures. Does the loss of consciousness define complex partial seizures in an otherwise what seems to be 'simple partial' clinically?

## Question 98
What is the definition of accepted rather than complete control of seizures in both partial and generalized tonic clonic seizures?

## Question 99
In an otherwise normal adolescent patient with no history of drug or alcohol intake, is it recommended that anti-epileptic drugs be started after the first generalized tonic–clonic fit?

## Question 100
Do antiepileptic drugs decrease libido in the long term? If they do, what treatment is recommended?

## Question 101
I'd like to know the possibility of giving these drugs in epileptics: vincamine (Oxicebral), cinnarizine, piribedil (Trivastal) and pentoxyphylline (Trental). I'd like to know if they are contraindicated.

## Question 102
If an epileptic patient, treated with oxcarbazepine, develops a rash, should this drug be withdrawn or the dosage decreased and then increased gradually again?

## Question 103
Does a patient with refractory epilepsy benefit from acetazolamide?

## Question 104
What anti-epileptic drug is recommended for a child with epilepsy and co-morbid attention deficit hyperactivity disorder (ADHD)? Can Ritalin safely be used for treatment?

## Question 105
What is the difference in efficacy and pharmacokinetics between sodium valproate and valproic acid?

## Question 106
Is it safe to give valproic acid to infants below 12 months of age?

## Question 107
How many times must the liver transaminases (SGOT and SGPT) rise to justify a discontinuation of valproic acid therapy in children? Which of these enzymes is more sensitive and reliable in this situation?

## Question 108
1. Does valproic acid block the photosensitivity phenomenon in reflex epilepsy?
2. Can a patient with this photosensitivity be safely exposed to computer games or other photic stimuli when receiving valproic acid treatment?
3. Does the photosensitivity phenomenon occur in partial seizures?

## Question 109
1. Can an epileptic fit be induced in idiopathic and symptomatic focal epilepsy syndromes by flickering lights?
2. Is valproate effective against the photosensitive phenomenon (seizure induction by flickering light)?

## Question 110
How much time should one give before a loading dose of phenytoin is judged to be ineffective in controlling seizures and an alternative should be instituted?

## Question 111
What is the maintenance dose of phenytoin in seizures arising as a complication of chronic renal failure?

## Question 112
I know that the loading dose of phenytoin in status epilepticus is 20 mg/kg with an upper limit of 1000 mg but if the same situation arose as a complication of chronic renal failure (on regular dialysis), should this dose remain the same or be reduced? If reduced, what should the dose be?

## Question 113
1. What is the most effective antiepileptic for a patient with simple partial motor status epilepticus who is not responding to a loading dose of phenytoin?
2. How long does phenytoin, given in a loading dose, take to work?

## Question 114
Is valproate effective if given rectally in status epilepticus and, if so, what dose is recommended?

## Question 115
In simple partial motor status epilepticus, if the patient does not respond to diazepam and phenytoin, is it justifiable to proceed to anaesthetic medication?

## Question 116
What is the recommended upper limit dose of lamotrigine when combined with both carbamazepine and valproate?

## Question 117
Is a valproate–lamotrigine combination more effective than carbamazepine on its own against partial seizures?

## Question 118
Why is the incidence of parkinsonism less common in smokers?

## Question 119
Is it recommended to start the treatment of parkinsonism with dopamine agonists alone in elderly (over 60 years old) patients, and to delay using L-dopa until the disease has progressed much further? Is there a rationale for this protocol in younger patients?

## Question 120
Does amantadine increase the endogenous release of dopamine, thus aiding early treatment of parkinsonism?

## Question 121
A 25-year-old woman, pregnant in her second trimester, starts to experience chorea and bilateral ankle arthralgia but has no past history of rheumatic chorea. In the first hour, her erythrocyte sedimentation rate is 70. Could this be no more than chorea gravidarum?

## Question 122
Is valproate as equally effective as haloperidol in the treatment of chorea, in particular rheumatic chorea?

## Question 123

Does a lesion of Guillain–Mollaret's triangle in the brain stem cause a type of myoclonus other than symptomatic palatal myoclonus?

## Question 124

1. In West's syndrome, after the fits have been suppressed, for how long should treatment with adrenocorticotrophic hormone (ACTH) continue?
2. Does complete suppression of resistant infantile myoclonic jerks by ACTH characterize West's syndrome?

## Question 125

Are anticholinergics the first line of treatment for primary torsion dystonia?

## Question 126

Can multiple sclerosis (MS) be associated with lack of vitamin D, lack of sunlight or low fish/cod-liver oil in the diet? By looking at the epidemiology (none at the equator; more outside 40° latitude, both north and south; less on top of Swiss mountains than in the Swiss valleys; more in fishing coastal towns and in Eskimos) this seems to be very important.

Vitamin D modulates the immune system and active vitamin D given to rats with experimental MS (acute encephalomyelitis) lowers the monocyte count in cerebrospinal fluid (CSF) by 90% in 72 hours with return of power to their limbs. Japanese MS patients who ate plenty of fish were found to have vitamin-D-receptor pleomorphism. The staple grains and cereals (wheat, barley, oats) eaten in Scandinavian and northern European countries contain phytic acid, which blocks vitamin D absorption, and rice is the only cereal free of phytic acid.

Are there any studies where low vitamin D levels in blood are associated with MS relapse?

## Question 127

What are the diagnostic criteria of 'definitive' multiple sclerosis (MS) – as taught to a medical student? We have found different information from different sources.

## Question 128

How reliable is a CT-brain scan with contrast in showing MS lesions as enhancing lesions in the presence of a contraindication to use MRI?

## Question 129

Is magnetic resonance (MR) spectroscopy of value in differentiating multiple sclerosis from cerebral autosomal dominant arteriopathy with subcortical infarctions (CADASIL)?

### Question 130

Does hemiplegia due to multiple sclerosis present with hemiparesis rather than dense hemiplegia (which is more characteristic of a stroke)? Other than age, what are the clinical signs that would help differentiate between the two?

### Question 131

If a female patient with multiple sclerosis wants to become pregnant, what are the risks, family planning advice and treatment, etc? What is the best advice to give to her?

### Question 132

Is there a role for methotrexate and azathioprine in the treatment of remitting-relapsing multiple sclerosis?

### Question 133

Do steroids have a role in preventing or ameliorating the relapses in relapsing-remitting multiple sclerosis?

### Question 134

Has cyclophosphamide a role in decreasing the rate and number of relapses in relapsing-remitting multiple sclerosis?

### Question 135

Is there evidence of the efficacy of cyclic pulse cyclophosphamide therapy in the treatment of relapsing-remitting multiple sclerosis?

### Question 136

Glatiramer acetate and interferon-beta are recommended by some people for the treatment of multiple sclerosis. Which drug should I use for a patient with a 2-year history of relapsing-remitting MS.

### Question 137

1. Most neurological books available to me say that high-dose IV dexamethasone can be used in acute relapses of multiple sclerosis (MS). What is the recommended dosage and regimen for this drug?
2. I understand that depot preparations of betamethasone (Depofos) can also be used in acute relapses of MS, as well as treatment for idiopathic Bell's palsy. If so, can you tell me the recommended dosage and regimen for this drug?

### Question 138

What are the most common causes of chronic meningitis and what investigations must be done?

## Question 139
What is Hib meningitis?

## Question 140
How often is tuberculosis a cause of chronic meningitis in comparison to other causes?

## Question 141
Is cavernous sinus thrombosis a complication of meningitis?

## Question 142
What is the mechanism of paraparesis that comes as a late (i.e. post-resolution) complication to meningitis?

## Question 143
Is lumbar puncture contraindicated in meningococcal meningitis?

## Question 144
What should the cerebrospinal fluid (CSF) picture be when the treatment of acute bacterial meningitis is complete, and after how many days of treatment?

## Question 145
In the management of meningococcaemia, can chloramphenicol be used as an alternative? Are there any advantages practically? The book quotes benzylpenicillin or cefotaxime (alternative). Are they a standard regimen?

## Question 146
'The immediate management of suspected meningococcal meningitis infection is benzylpenicillin 1200 mg either by slow IV injection or intramuscularly, prior to investigations.'
   Is this always true? Should you not perform a lumbar puncture for culture first?

## Question 147
Should children with bacterial meningitis be treated with steroids to prevent complications?

## Question 148
What is the role of anticonvulsants in a case of encephalitis and how long should one continue them?

## Question 149
How effective are steroids in the treatment of radiculomyelitis?

## Question 150
Should you treat a patient who has a brain cysticercosis lesion? The text seems to say 'Yes' but there is great uncertainty about it.
Also, should one 'worm' the patient's gut when you find brain lesions; if so, with what?

## Question 151
Is there any rationale for giving either propranolol, valproate or buspirone to patients with cerebellar ataxia?

## Question 152
Is there a laboratory marker for cerebral dominant arteriopathy with subcortical infarcts and leucoencephalopathy (CADASIL)? Is serum lactic acid elevated?

## Question 153
Primary brain tumours rarely metastasize outside the brain but malignancies outside the brain frequently metastasize to the brain. Why?

## Question 154
In a case of brain tumour, can papilloedema occur without a headache?

## Question 155
What are the pathological diagnostic features of glioblastoma multiforme?

## Question 156
Is acetazolamide effective in cases of normal pressure hydrocephalus? How effective is low-dose digoxin?

## Question 157
If dementia and incontinence are present, but gait apraxia is not, can normal pressure hydrocephalus be diagnosed?

## Question 158
Is a normal CT (plain and with contrast) in patients with headache, bilateral papilloedema and a clear conscious level sufficient to diagnose benign intracranial hypertension?

## Question 159
What is the value above which cerebrospinal fluid (CSF) pressure is said to be raised?

## Question 160
Could benign intracranial hypertension be diagnosed without headache as a complaint?

## Question 161
Can pyramidal tract lesions present as false localizing signs in benign intracranial hypertension?

## Question 162
How often can increased intracranial hypertension be present without papilloedema on examination?

## Question 163
Which is the most effective method of reducing raised intracranial pressure: mannitol, steroids or ventilation?

## Question 164
In the case of pseudotumour cerebri, if this is proved to be due to sagittal sinus thrombosis with no explanation for the thrombosis, should the patient receive lifelong anticoagulation treatment?

## Question 165
Does digitalis help reduce cerebrospinal fluid (CSF) formation, specifically in the treatment of resistant benign intracranial hypertension?

## Question 166
Is it safe to combine hydrochlorothiazide, amiloride, acetazolamide and digitalis (125 μg per day) in a hypertensive patient with idiopathic intracranial hypertension (pseudotumour cerebri)?

## Question 167
What is the best indicator for monitoring the efficacy of treatment or the progress of the disease in pseudotumor cerebri? Is it by the disappearance of papilloedema, the relief of headache or by frequent visual field examination or cerebrospinal fluid (CSF) pressure?

## Question 168
What is the definition of 'bursting' when describing a headache?

## Question 169
1. What drugs, other than tricyclic antidepressants, can be used in prophylaxis for daily tension headache?
2. Is propranolol an effective treatment?

## Question 170
Are maprotiline and imipramine as effective as amitriptyline in the treatment of tension headache?

## Question 171
How often does migraine headache present unilaterally?

## Question 172
Are ergotamine-containing preparations contraindicated in the treatment of resistant migraine in hypertensive patients? Can I give it, under close supervision of the blood pressure, in the emergency room?

## Question 173
Should ergotamine be given to abort a migrainous attack in a pregnant female? If not, what is the recommended alternative?

## Question 174
What is the frequency of migrainous attacks above which prophylactic therapy should be commenced? If commenced, for how long should the treatment be continued and what should be done if frequent attacks recur after discontinuation of the prophylactic treatment?

## Question 175
Is verapamil more effective in migraine prophylaxis than flunarizine?

## Question 176
Are imipramine and fluoxetine effective as a prophylactic treatment against migraine? Are they as effective as amitriptyline?

## Question 177
1. Is sodium valproate more effective than valproic acid with regard to migraine prophylaxis and anti-epileptic activity?
2. Is carbamazepine effective as a prophylaxis against migraine?

## Question 178
Can flunarizine, diltiazem and nifedipine be used in the treatment of a cluster headache and do they have the same efficacy as verapamil?

## Question 179
If cluster headache migraine is confidently diagnosed in general practice, is it worth trying lithium prophylaxis or should this commence at secondary care level? Which other treatment is recommended?

## Question 180
Is ergotamine effective in preventing an attack of cluster headache?

## Question 181
In the case of anterior spinal artery occlusion is bladder function preserved or is there urine retention?

**Question 182**
In the case of anterior spinal artery occlusion, can the patient have intact sensations in the lower limbs?

**Question 183**
In the case of anterior spinal artery occlusion, will the paraplegia be of a spastic or a flaccid type?

**Question 184**
Can fasciculations occur in radiculopathy or peripheral neuropathy or is it pathognomonic to anterior horn cell lesion?

**Question 185**
Is ibuprofen recommended in prophylaxis or treatment of Alzheimer's dementia?

**Question 186**
What are the principal causes of frontotemporal dementia and how can the cause be diagnosed?

**Question 187**
What are the associated features of meningomyelocele other than hydrocephalus, urinary incontinence and paraplegia? Do patients have congenital heart disease and congenital dislocation of hips?

**Question 188**
Can a patient with neurofibromatosis type I have a neurofibroma arising from a nerve root or radicle causing cervical or compressive lumbar radiculopathy?

**Question 189**
Is there a way to retard the rate of development of cutaneous or other manifestations of neurofibromatosis type 1? Has a cure for this condition yet been found?

**Question 190**
How does neurofibromatosis type 2 (NF2) affect the heart?

**Question 191**
1. How often is leprosy a cause of mononeuritis multiplex?
2. How often is diabetes mellitus a cause of mononeuritis multiplex?

**Question 192**
What is the expected response of straight leg-raising if the meningeal stretch test is positive? Is it back pain, pain in the sciatic distribution, or limitation in the range of leg-raising?

## Question 193

1. Does radiculopathy due to systemic disease produce positive meningeal stretch signs or are these limited to radiculopathy as a result of disc prolapse?
2. Where no cause is found for radiculopathy, is steroid treatment indicated?

## Question 194

What are the most common causes of radiculopathy?

## Question 195

1. Does the absence of a positive straight leg-raising test exclude radiculopathy?
2. Can radiculopathy be diagnosed by meningeal stretch tests or is it diagnosed electrophysiologically?

## Question 196

Why does ascending paralysis occur in the Guillain–Barré syndrome?

## Question 197

Is systemic steroid therapy indicated in cases of carpal tunnel syndrome not responsive to conservative measures?

## Question 198

Is there a role for acetazolamide in the treatment of carpal tunnel syndrome? What is the dose? How can paraesthesia induced by the drug be overcome?

## Question 199

Can an MRI scan of the cervical spine detect cervical rib or does this merit an individual scan?

## Question 200

Please explain the mechanism by which cervical spondylosis causes acroparaesthesia without proximal sensory affection. Does this happen by compromising the blood supply?

## Question 201

Can chronic inflammatory demyelinating polyradiculoneuropathy be associated with positive stretch tests such as Lasègue's sign?

## Question 202

1. If a patient with a spastic paraplegia due to a spinal cord lesion is able to sit unaided, does this indicate intact dorsal segments (T7–T12)?

2. What mechanism underlies the inability of some patients with spastic paraplegia to sit in bed with their lower limbs straight on the bed, while able to sit on the edge of the bed with their lower limbs hanging?

### Question 203
What is the scientific definition of asthenia and weakness?

### Question 204
Why do the following cause weakness that is more proximal than distal:
- Muscle disease.
- Radiculopathy.
- Anterior horn cell disease.

### Question 205
What is the difference between fibrillation, fasciculations and myokymia?

### Question 206
What is the difference between 'Isaac's syndrome' and 'stiff person syndrome'?

### Question 207
What is the most common cause for fibrosis of the quadriceps femoris muscle?

### Question 208
In a patient receiving long-term oral steroids and gradually developing proximal muscle weakness, how does one differentiate between steroid myopathy and myositis?

### Question 209
What is viral myositis?

### Question 210
Does myositis affect the facial and neck muscles?

### Question 211
I am a neurologist and would like to know:
- What precautions I should take with regard to the cardiovascular system, before and after prescribing mexiletine for cases of myotonia.
- Whether there is a group of patients who should not receive this drug.

### Question 212
Can myasthenia gravis be unilateral and, if so, how often?

## Question 213
Can the creatine phosphokinase (CPK) level in the blood, or the presence of certain auto-antibodies, help to differentiate muscle dystrophies from myositis?

## Question 214
Can percussion myotonia occur with motor neurone disease? If so, please explain the mechanism and cause–effect for this.

## Question 215
Can benign intracranial hypertension be diagnosed on the basis of persistent headache and CT-brain scan findings of slit ventricles with no papilloedema and preserved spontaneous venous pulsations on ophthalmoscopy? And do you recommend cerebrospinal fluid (CSF) pressure measurement as a routine investigation in the diagnosis of this type of disorder?

## Question 216
In my experience in the treatment of stroke patients, the combination of atenolol 50 mg, hydrochlorothiazide 25 mg and amlodipine 10 mg is very effective in the treatment of resistant hypertension. Can you tell me whether this combination of antihypertensives is contraindicated in diabetic patients?

## Question 217
Can diabetic mononeuropathy of the third cranial nerve cause ipsilateral pain of the face and tenderness (but not redness) of the affected eye? Can these symptoms be explained by Tolosa–Hunt syndrome?

## Question 218
1. For how long should adrenocorticotrophic hormone (ACTH) be given to patients after stoppage of myoclonic seizures in West's syndrome?
2. If seizures recur after stoppage, should ACTH be re-administered?

## Question 219
In acute attacks of multiple sclerosis (MS), where methylprednisolone is not available, can pulse steroid therapy be given with a one-off dose of 200 mg dexamethasone?

## Question 220
Is there a role for aciclovir in idiopathic Bell's palsy?

## Question 221
Does temporal arteritis headache or other pain respond to non-steroidal anti-inflammatory drugs?

## Question 222
What is the recommended target of total and low-density lipoprotein (LDL) cholesterol in secondary prevention of ischaemic stroke?

## Question 223
Is intravenous sodium nitroprusside contraindicated in lowering resistant hypertension secondary to primary intracerebral haemorrhage?

## Question 224
After how long can a patient with primary intracerebral haemorrhage safely be prescribed aspirin for secondary prophylaxis of further ischemic strokes? Or should aspirin no longer be prescribed in this case?

## Question 225
Does occlusion of the recurrent Heubner's artery result in weakness of the upper limb that is proximal more than distal?

## Question 226
I have recently been told by fellow cardiologists that statins have a role to play in the acute management of myocardial infarction: is this true? And does this extend to the acute management of ischemic stroke?

## Question 227
What is captocormia?

## ANSWERS

### Answer 1
Sharp brief pains often occur for no known reason. Nerve entrapment is said to be one cause, without much evidence.

### Answer 2
Foot drop with loss of eversion and dorsiflexion of the foot occurs when the common peroneal nerve is injured at the head of the fibula (e.g. from fracture or from compression by a leg plaster). The nerve is very superficial at this point. Prolonged crossing of the legs, particularly in an emaciated person, is a further cause. It can also occur in diseases affecting the peripheral nerves and motor neurones in the spinal cord.

### Answer 3
Abnormal sensations, often tingling or painful, occurring with minimal stimulation.

### Answer 4
There is no difference; most use the term 'light touch', which is used to test sensation via the posterior columns.

### Answer 5
Apraxia means loss of ability to perform a function despite no sensory or motor abnormalities; in this case loss of ability to walk. It is due to bilateral frontal lesions. Brun's syndrome is due to an intermittent blockage of the aqueduct of Sylvius, usually due to a brain tumour. Apraxia is one of the signs of this syndrome.

### Answer 6
When eliciting the plantar reflex the stick should run along the outer edge of the sole of the foot from the heel towards the little toe. Babinski did not use a medial movement across the sole of the foot.

### Answer 7
Dopamine agonists are not of value in aphasic patients.

### Answer 8
They have no confirmed role.

### Answer 9
The VIth nerve nucleus sends axons directly into the VIth nerve to supply the lateral rectus, and also into the contralateral medial longitudinal fasciculus and up into the IIIrd nerve nucleus where they

synapse with neurones from the medial rectus. Damage to the VIth nerve nucleus prevents both eyes moving ipsilaterally. A bilateral VIth nerve palsy is always a false localizing sign.

## Answer 10
The term 'incongruous homonymous hemianopia' is used for lesions in the optic tracts or chiasm. The word homonymous can only be used when the same half of both fields of vision is lost.

## Answer 11
Optic neuritis is usually due to a demyelinating process, most commonly multiple sclerosis. Treatment is usually not required.

## Answer 12
This is highly likely to be multiple sclerosis (MS) and MRI shows lesions in 85% of patients with clinical MS. Time will tell.

## Answer 13
You might find that reducing the background illumination will help, with patient fixating a distant object.

## Answer 14
Interruption of the oculomotor nerve abolishes the light reflex on the side of the lesion; the reflex (consensual) stays in the other eye. Damage to the retina or optic nerve causes absent light reflex in both eyes when light is shone into the eye on the side of the lesion.

## Answer 15
Yes, trigeminal neuralgia can occur in, for example multiple sclerosis and tumours of the 5th nerve.

## Answer 16
Usually, yes. The maximum dose is 1.6 g daily.

## Answer 17
Yes, although there are no good controlled trials.

## Answer 18
Combination therapy, e.g. carbamazepine with phenytoin, baclofen or gabapentin.

## Answer 19
Recurrent facial palsy is rare; it is usually idiopathic. It is called Melkersson's syndrome.

## Answer 20
Taste is not affected in supranuclear lesions (i.e. upper motor neurone lesions). Involvement of the facial nerve proximal to the origin of the chorda tympani will cause loss of taste. Lesions beyond the stylomastoid foramen will not affect taste.

## Answer 21
No. Synacthen (tetracosactide) is an analogue of corticotrophin (adrenocorticotrophin hormone; ACTH). It is only used in stimulation tests to assess adrenocortical function.

## Answer 22
Trials are not conclusive, but aciclovir with steroids (prednisolone 60 mg daily initially) might be beneficial and is the most common current therapy.

## Answer 23
Yes.

## Answer 24
No these drugs are not very effective in this type of vertigo.

## Answer 25
Yes; methylprednisolone alone is as effective as is the combination of methylprednisolone and valaciclovir, and better than valaciclovir alone. More trials are needed, but it is reasonable to use steroids.

## Answer 26
Fortunately we can overcome any gag reflex that is present when we swallow.

## Answer 27
Head nodding is due to a basal ganglia lesion not a cerebellar lesion. It does occur without features of parkinsonism.

## Answer 28
1. Valproate is sometimes used, particularly when the myoclonus is related to epilepsy.
2. Yes.

## Answer 29
Yes, if sustained. Unsustained ankle clonus can occur normally.

## Answer 30
Providing there is no marked weakness of the outstretched limbs, pronator drift is pathognomonic of a pyramidal lesion.

## Answer 31
The weakness often starts distally, e.g. the hands, but then spreads to involve forearms, the biceps and triceps followed by shoulder muscles.

## Answer 32
Proximal weakness can occur with a pyramidal tract lesion.

## Answer 33
This is a question of terminology. Brisk reflexes, to most clinicians, mean slightly exaggerated reflexes as seen in an anxious person. Hyperreflexia usually implies a pathological increase, i.e. an upper motor neurone (UMN) lesion.

## Answer 34
Pyramidal lesions sometimes produce only minor degrees of weakness accompanied by loss of skilful movements. In Wartenberg's reflex the patient is asked to flex the terminal phalanges of the fingers of one hand against the flexed fingers of the examiner. On striking the back of the examiner's fingers with a patellar hammer, the thumb remains extended and abducted in normals. Following a pyramidal lesion (corticospinal tract) the thumb adducts and flexes. This sign would only be very suggestive but not diagnostic of a pyramidal lesion; it is not often used.

## Answer 35
An extensor plantar response is a valuable sign in diagnosing a pyramidal tract lesion. However, it can sometimes be difficult to elicit, and in the presence of typical weakness and pathological reflexes a pyramidal lesion can still be diagnosed.

## Answer 36
No; it is not common and investigation (cerebral CT or MRI) is required. Incidentally, it is better to use the term extensor plantar response rather than Babinski (which was described in babies).

## Answer 37
This is not a reliable observation. Remember the cord ends at L1, so a paraplegia by definition must occur with a lesion above this and below the cervical region.

## Answer 38
Brown–Séquard syndrome – hemisection of the cord – gives ipsilateral diminished proprioception and vibration sense and weakness, with contralateral decrease in pain and temperature sensation (because of crossing of the fibres of the spinothalamic tract). A small lesion in, for example, MS may give ipsilateral weakness and diminished sensation only. It is not strictly the Brown–Séquard syndrome.

## Answer 39

*Method 1*
With the patient's arm flexed to a right angle, the patient is then asked to pronate and supinate the forearm as rapidly as possible. Normal is rapid with no jerking; with dysdiadochokinesis, movements are slow and irregular.

*Method 2*
The patient is asked to tap the examiner's palm with the fingertips alternating in supination and pronation as fast as possible. This is irregular and slow in dysdiadochokinesis. If the tapping is done onto a hard surface, the sound will also be irregular.

## Answer 40

Kinetic and intention tremors are the same.

## Answer 41

Treatment is unsatisfactory. Try propranolol, primidone or piracetam.

## Answer 42

When the biceps and supinator reflexes are brisk this might be accompanied by finger flexion. Sometimes, however, finger flexion still occurs with depression of the direct reflex and this is called inversion. It is due to a lesion at C5–C6, which interrupts the reflex arc but if it compresses the corticospinal tract as well it will give exaggerated reflexes in lower segments (i.e. C7–C8 – finger flexion). An inverted knee jerk occurs with a lesion at L2–L4.

## Answer 43

Allodynia is an abnormal sensory experience (usually painful) to a normal stimulus. Patients with posterior column lesions do not suffer with allodynia.

## Answer 44

In patients with neuropathic pain, carbamazepine is still first-line therapy. Gabapentin is effective in painful diabetic neuropathy and post-herpetic neuralgia.

## Answer 45

Dissociative means dissociation between posterior column sensation (light touch, vibration) and spinothalamic tracts (pain and temperature). These can be tested, e.g. with cotton wool and a sterile pin.

## Answer 46

Any non-ionic monomeric contrast agent can be used. The dose is equivalent of 15 g iodine.

## Answer 47
Use 300 mg iodine/mL dosage. Give 50 mL 10 minutes before the procedure.

## Answer 48
1. On T2-weighted images, tissue with short T2 decay times (fat) appears dark, while tissues with long T2 decay times (water) appear bright. FLAIR is used, for example, to suppress the high cerebrospinal fluid signal in T2 so that lesions can be seen more clearly.
2. Magnetization transfer coherence is a technique to increase the contrast-to-noise ratio between normal and pathological tissues.

## Answer 49
It refers to lumbosacral spines.

## Answer 50
Squeezing the Achilles tendon and rubbing the front of the chest hard are two common stimuli. Try to be consistent for comparison.

## Answer 51
With difficulty! Do your best.

## Answer 52
Loss of consciousness occurs but is rare. It usually occurs in TIAs affecting the posterior circulation. The mechanism is inhibition of the ascending reticular activating system.

## Answer 53
Surgery is recommended in TIA and stroke patients when stenosis narrows the carotid lumen by more than 70%; but not in patients with a total stenosis.

## Answer 54
Stenosis of the carotid artery by greater than 70% should be managed surgically or by placing a stent.

## Answer 55
No.

## Answer 56
Medulla and brainstem, but the anatomy is not clear.

## Answer 57
The symptoms of vertebrobasilar insufficiency can be vague, e.g. dizziness, which might be associated with hyperventilation, which can lead to circumoral numbness.

## Answer 58

Wallenberg, in his original description of the lateral medullary infarction syndrome, did not include diplopia. Diplopia does occur; remember that the VIth nerve is very near to the Vth nerve nucleus.

*Further reading*
Fisher CM et al. (1961) Lateral medullary infarction – the pattern of vascular occlusion. *Journal of Neuropathology and Experimental Neurology* **20**: 323.

## Answer 59

Hypotonia is a feature of an acute upper motor neurone lesion, which may last for several days. This is replaced by hypertonia due to loss of the inhibiting effects of the corticospinal pathways.

## Answer 60

Most patients with TIAs do not lose consciousness and also are not seen in hospital. Because the episodes last less than 24 hours it is usually something that you get from the history. However, a CT/MRI scan is mandatory to rule out haemorrhage so that thrombolytic therapy can be started. Remember, an infarction will only be detected later.

*Further reading*
Chalela JA et al. (2007) MRI and CT in emergency assessment of patients with suspected acute stroke. *Lancet* **369**: 293–298.

## Answer 61

You do this by referring to the anatomical diagrams in the book *(see K&C 6e, p. 1192)*.

*Examples*
A common lesion from a CVA is due to a thrombosis in the middle cerebral artery in the internal capsule, as shown in Fig. 21.8. Damage to the left pyramidal tract at this position produces a right hemiplegia (the tracts have already crossed) with upper motor neurone signs (Table 21.12) in the face, right arm and leg. The left side of the cortex is also affected by a thrombus in the middle cerebral artery and this would produce aphasia [see Fig. 21.2 (p.1177)]. When a lesion occurs in the brainstem, not only is the pyramidal tract involved (see Fig. 21.8) but cranial nerves will also be affected, depending on exactly where the lesion is [see Fig. 21.7 (p. 1185)]. It is by knowing the neuroanatomy that clinicians can correlate the signs with the site of the lesion.

*Further reading*
Patten J (1996) *Neurological Differential Diagnosis*, 7th edn. London: Springer-Verlag.

## Answer 62

Patients with a carotid artery dissection are often treated with anticoagulants despite the underlying bleeding into the vessel wall. As the blood enters the wall of the artery the lumen becomes progressively narrowed and thrombosed. It is to try to prevent further thrombosis and emboli occurring that anticoagulants are given.

## Answer 63

Heparin can be used in patients not suitable (because of lapse in time or risks) for thrombolysis but the data on benefit are scant. Aspirin is of benefit. On the whole heparin is not recommended. Active thromboplastin time (APTT) is used for monitoring heparin therapy.

## Answer 64

In general no, but occasionally heparin has been used in patients with recurrent transient ischaemic attacks on antiplatelet therapy.

## Answer 65

1. No; heparin is not used in most stroke cases. Studies with LMWH have shown similar results to unfractionated heparin.
2. In one trial, 7 days. At 3 months there was no benefit.

## Answer 66

No, streptokinase is not now used as altepase is preferred. Dose is 0.9 mg/kg (maximum 90 mg).

*Further reading*
Wahlgren N et al. (2007) Thrombolysis for acute ischaemic stroke (SITS-MOST). *Lancet* **369**: 275–282.

## Answer 67

The CAST study, which involved over 21 000 patients, showed a clear benefit of aspirin for acute ischaemic strokes. Because of this, it is now recommended that aspirin be given to all patients who are not eligible for thrombolytic (altepase) therapy. Accurate CT or MRI can rule out haemorrhage quickly so that aspirin can be used.

## Answer 68

The evidence is inconclusive. CT/MRI must always be performed to rule out haemorrhage. Aspirin is probably just as good; the combination better, but with a higher risk of haemorrhage.

## Answer 69

There is little rationale for this treatment although it is sometimes advocated for recurrent strokes, particularly transient ischaemic attacks.

## Answer 70

1. There may be some value in the dipyridamol–aspirin combination but there is no very good evidence of efficacy and this adds to the expense of therapy.

2. No, there is no evidence that aspirin plus anticoagulant combination is superior to antiplatelet therapy.

## Answer 71

1. Yes it is safe. There is no good evidence of neuroprotective effect.
2. Yes it is safe but it is probably wiser to use atenolol or amlodipine, which have been more widely used.
3. Neither are of real help.

## Answer 72

Tracking of blood beneath the retinal hyaloid membrane. CSF does not gain access to the subhyaloid space.

## Answer 73

- Prevention: nimodipine 60 mg orally (or by nasogastric tube). This should be given every 4 hours starting within 4 days of haemorrhage. Give for 21 days.
- Treatment: intravenous infusion into central veins, initially 1 mg/hour increasing to 2 mg/hour if no fall in blood pressure. Continue for 5–10 days and at least 5 days after surgery.

*Further reading*
Van Gijn J et al. (2007). Subarachnoid haemorrhage. *Lancet* **369**: 306–318.

## Answer 74

No, allopurinol should not be given to stroke patients.

## Answer 75

There is, of course, a causal link between atherosclerosis and ischaemic stroke. Hyperuricaemia is often seen in obese, diabetic, hypertensive patients, particularly if they drink excess alcohol. It is not causal.

## Answer 76

No. They are not helpful.

## Answer 77

Valproate is only useful if the myoclonus is part of the epileptic syndrome. L-dopa is not usually of benefit.

## Answer 78

This is very difficult as thrombolytic therapy is completely out of the question. Angioplasty with stenting might be an option but this usually requires antiplatelet therapy, which would be contraindicated. All in all, a patient such as you describe would not be a good-risk candidate.

## Answer 79
There are a few well-constructed randomized controlled trials (RCTs) in this condition. Heparin is given in standard doses but the evidence for its value is small. It is followed by warfarin and heparin is stopped when the international normalized ratio is in the target range of 2.5.

*Further reading*
Stam J (2005) Thrombosis of the cerebral veins and sinuses. *New England Journal of Medicine* **352**: 1791–1798.

## Answer 80
Possibly for 1 year.

*Further reading*
Stam J (2005) Thrombosis of the cerebral veins and sinuses. *New England Journal of Medicine* **352**: 1791–1798.

## Answer 81
Seizures occur in 3% of hospitalized acute-stroke patients, usually those with a large cortical infarct or haemorrhage. Recurrence rates after first seizures are higher in groups with vascular disease than within idiopathic epilepsy.

*Further reading*
Shinton R et al. (1988) The frequency, characteristics and prognosis of epileptic seizures at the onset of stroke. *Journal of Neurology, Neurosurgery, and Psychiatry* **51**: 273.

## Answer 82
Epilepsy in the first week after a cerebrovascular accident does not usually lead to persistence. Drugs could be withdrawn after about 6 months.

## Answer 83
During a seizure, the EEG is almost invariably abnormal because spikes reach the brain surface. Many people with epilepsy have a normal EEG between fits and thus a normal EEG between attacks is of no help in diagnosis. Similarly, mild EEG abnormalities are not uncommon in the general population and should not in themselves be used to diagnose epilepsy.

Metabolic brain disorders, e.g. hepatic encephalopathy, give specific EEG abnormalities but again are not helpful in the diagnosis of epilepsy.

Whenever antiepileptic drugs are withdrawn there is a risk that the patient will have another epileptic attack; this is not due to the drugs.

## Answer 84
Uncinate fits are characterized by an olfactory or gustatory aura often with motor movement, e.g. licking lips.

**Answer 85**
Epilepsy during sleep is not pathognomonic for any particular epileptic syndrome.

**Answer 86**
An organic pathology is possible. It must be distinguished from postictal automatism following sleep seizures and from complex partial seizures. An abnormal EEG would help in the diagnosis.

**Answer 87**
These are not usual in tonic–clonic fits. They occur more often in a complex partial seizure in the period of behavioural arrest before the ictal phase.

**Answer 88**
It is very uncommon.

**Answer 89**
In partial seizures arising from the temporal lobe, auras are common. They can be visual (flashing lights) or olfactory (smell), for example.

**Answer 90**
'Pseudoseizures' is the term used for seizures that appear to be epileptic but are not. 'Pseudo-pseudoseizures' is a term occasionally used to suggest a psychogenic cause.

**Answer 91**
No, delay does not result in more frequent seizures.

**Answer 92**
Genetic disorder accounts for less than 1% of patients with epilepsy and tests are not recommended. Mutation analysis is available for suspected Huntington's disease but should only be performed by designated centres.

**Answer 93**
Despite its limitations, an EEG is still worthwhile doing after a first fit. It might be useful to show an abnormality, which helps to confirm the diagnosis. A normal EEG, however, does not exclude epilepsy (*see K&C 6e, p. 1222*). Once a diagnosis is established, further EEGs are not required.

**Answer 94**
'Drop attacks', by definition, result in the patient falling to the ground, but there is no loss of consciousness.

## Answer 95
They do not cause falls very often.

## Answer 96
The data favour complex partial seizures. Most patients with a haemoglobin of 10.8 g/dL are asymptomatic.

## Answer 97
Yes, loss of consciousness does differentiate between the two seizures. Loss of consciousness occurs in complex partial seizures, but not in simple.

## Answer 98
Twenty per cent of patients with epilepsy still have seizures despite good therapy. In these patients, this is the best that can be done so is 'accepted'. Complete control means no seizures or seizures very rarely.

## Answer 99
Patients who have a low risk of recurrence are those with a normal electroencephalogram, no history of head injury, normal brain imaging and no family history. These patients can be left untreated after the first seizure if they are carefully counselled and know exactly what to expect. However, there is a 40% risk of a further seizure. They must not drive for 1 year.

## Answer 100
Not usually, although it has been reported with carbamazepine. Ethosuximide increases libido. Treatment is with phosphodiesterase type-5 inhibitors, e.g. sildenafil.

## Answer 101
Vincamine (a natural substance derived from the *Vinca minor* plant; a vasodilator) and piribedil (a dopamine agonist) are not available as drugs in the UK. Cinnarizine is not contraindicated but pentoxyfylline should not be given.

## Answer 102
The drug should be withdrawn as the rash is probably a hypersensitive reaction. It is better to change to another drug.

## Answer 103
Acetazolamide has been used with carbamazepine in refractory cases.

### Further reading
Oles KS et al. (1989) Use of acetazolamide as an adjunct to carbamazepine in refractory partial seizures. *Epilepsia* **30**: 74–78.

## Answer 104
There is no one drug in this situation. It partly depends on the type of epilepsy. Any drug must be used carefully. Either valproate or ethosuximide is a reasonable choice but both are associated with hyperactivity. Do not use Ritalin.

## Answer 105
None: pharmacokinetic studies show absorption, distribution and protein binding to be similar.

## Answer 106
Hepatotoxicity is more common in children under 2 years. Close supervision is required, particularly if multiple drugs are being used.

## Answer 107
SGOT (serum glutamic oxaloacetic transaminase) (or AST (aspartate transferase)) and SGPT (serum glutamic pyruvic transaminase) (or ALT (Alanine transferase)) are often transiently raised, usually in the first 6 months of therapy. Prothrombin time (a measure of liver function) is a useful guide to therapy, and valproate should be stopped if prothrombin time is prolonged.

## Answer 108
1. Valproic acid is used in reflex epilepsy.
2. Yes; providing the fits have been controlled and are not induced by the photic stimuli.
3. Yes.

## Answer 109
1. Yes.
2. Valproate is effective, but less so than when used for generalized seizures. Carbamazepine is probably first choice.

## Answer 110
Phenytoin has a narrow therapeutic index. The time to peak concentration after an oral dose of phenytoin is 4–12 hours with a half-life of 9–140 hours. This implies a long time with measurements of the blood level of phenytoin to check whether they are in the therapeutic range.

## Answer 111
Usually 150–300 mg with plasma phenytoin monitoring.

## Answer 112
The dose is the same.

## Answer 113
1. Carbamazepine is a good choice.
2. Up to 30 minutes.

## Answer 114
Valproate is not recommended for rectal use.

## Answer 115
The patient is conscious in simple partial motor status epilepticus. If initially refractory to diazepam and phenytoin, care in an ITU is required, with repeat of the initial therapy. Anaesthetic medication would be the last resort and only with good anaesthetic and monitoring facilities.

## Answer 116
Carbamazepine is an enzyme inducer and tends to reduce blood levels of lamotrigine; valproate increases the levels. Monotherapy is best if possible.

Dose: lamotrigine 100–200 mg daily with valproate; 200–400 mg without valproate.

## Answer 117
Carbamazepine is the drug of choice; valproate–lamotrigine is only second-line therapy. Remember, valproate increases the plasma lamotrigine concentration and therefore dose reduction might well be required with this combination.

## Answer 118
It is quite true that parkinsonism is much less common in smokers. There is no obvious reason for this.

## Answer 119
Because of the major distressing side-effects of L-dopa therapy over time, it is now thought that treatment with L-dopa should be delayed as long as possible in all age groups. It does not alter the natural progression of Parkinson's disease.

## Answer 120
Yes, Amantadine stimulates the release of dopamine stored in nerve terminals. It also reduces re-uptake of released dopamine by the presynaptic neurone.

## Answer 121
You must exclude other causes, e.g. rheumatic fever, antiphospholipid syndrome, Wilson's disease and ingestion of toxic substances. Chorea gravidarum does, however, occur in the second trimester.

## Answer 122
Diazepam is usually used in Sydenham's (rheumatic) chorea. Dopamine antagonists are next in line. Valproate has no proven effect.

## Answer 123
Central tegmental olivary lesions occur which can be the result of vascular, neoplastic or traumatic injury. Symptomless palatal myoclonus is rare; no other type of myoclonus occurs with this lesion.

## Answer 124
'Infantile spasms' occur in West's syndrome:
1. The length of time to give ACTH is uncertain but 2 weeks has been used in many studies. A further course is given for relapses.
2. No; response can be as low as 40%, although 80% is a more usual figure.

## Answer 125
They should be called antimuscarinics and, yes, they are first-choice therapy.

## Answer 126
As the questioner points out, there is a lot of epidemiological data on MS and there has been an inevitable link with sunlight and vitamin D.

A quick search reveals no studies of low blood levels of vitamin D (25-hydroxycholecalciferol) and relapse in MS, but the Multiple Sclerosis Society (http://www.mssociety.org.uk), might be able to help.

## Answer 127
The diagnostic criteria depend on the clinical demonstration of a lesion in the CNS that is disseminated in time and space. The first episode might be localized and only time will make the diagnosis clear when another lesion in another place occurs. MRI is fairly sensitive but not specific.

## Answer 128
Not reliable; MRI is the gold standard.

## Answer 129
CADASIL is rare but characteristic findings are seen in the subcortical white matter. MR findings in multiple sclerosis are usually periventricular. However, this is not entirely specific on its own but usually with the clinical picture (dissemination of symptoms and signs in time and position) the diagnosis can be reached.

## Answer 130
Hemiparesis, rather than a dense hemiplegia, would be more likely in MS but remember to be careful in making a diagnosis of MS if the signs are not disseminated in time and space. This is how you differentiate MS clinically from other conditions, plus an MRI for confirmation.

## Answer 131
There have been many studies, with an impression that the risk of a relapse of the disease is slightly increased in pregnancy, particularly in the puerperium. There is no evidence that pregnancy affects the long-term prognosis, and most clinicians no longer advise against pregnancy.

## Answer 132
Randomized controlled trials of methotrexate have shown no benefit. Meta-analysis of seven trials with azathioprine has shown a slight benefit but this is offset by the side-effects.

## Answer 133
No, steroids have no role in the prevention of relapses but they are used when a relapse occurs.

## Answer 134
It has been used in small trials but there is no overall effect.

## Answer 135
Small clinical trials have been performed with no consistent evidence of efficacy.

## Answer 136
Both drugs have been approved by the US Food and Drug Administration for relapsing-remitting MS. You can use either as first choice but they are expensive.

## Answer 137
1. The best studies use IV methylprednisolone 1 g per day for 3 days.
2. Bell's palsy can be helped by steroids; use prednisolone combined with aciclovir.

## Answer 138
The common causes are tuberculosis and fungal, e.g. cryptoococcal. Sarcoidosis, syphilis and Behçet's syndrome can also cause chronic meningitis (see K&C 6e, p. 1238). Lumbar puncture is the most valuable investigation.

## Answer 139
Meningitis caused by *Haemophilus influenzae* type b (Hib). This is now rare in countries where the Hib vaccine is available.

## Answer 140
No exact figures are easily available as frequency depends, for example, on which country, co-infection with HIV and many other factors.

TB meningitis is, however, quite a common cause of meningitis and must always be high on the list of possible causes.

## Answer 141
No, cavernous sinus thrombosis is not a complication, although cortical vein thrombosis is. The CSF is usually abnormal in cavernous sinus thrombosis, which may be a cause of confusion.

## Answer 142
This is rare; the mechanism is unclear.

## Answer 143
In a case of meningococcal meningitis and a purpuric rash, lumbar puncture is not necessary and can be dangerous. If there is doubt about the diagnosis and no evidence of a mass lesion on CT/MRI, lumbar puncture should be performed.

## Answer 144
It is not usual to repeat the lumbar puncture in acute bacterial meningitis but the findings should parallel the clinical condition. Antibiotics are usually given for 7–10 days and by then the CSF should be returning to normal.

## Answer 145
Chloramphenicol was used in meningococcaemia. It is often extremely effective but of course does have the disadvantage of, albeit rarely, causing aplastic anaemia. The treatment of choice is still penicillin with cefotaxime as an alternative. Chloramphenicol can be used in the severely beta-lactam-allergic patient.

## Answer 146
Yes, your statement is true. Primary care physicians should give penicillin as soon as possible in a suspected case of meningococcal meningitis. Minutes count in this disease. A lumbar puncture can be performed later.

## Answer 147
Meta-analysis shows no reduction in mortality but a reduction of neurological or hearing deficits if dexamethasone is given early at the time of the first antibiotic dose. There is, however, much debate on the subject. Dexamethasone should certainly be given to children with Hib meningitis.

## Answer 148

Any seizures that occur in a patient with encephalitis will need treatment which should be continued for approximately 3 months although there is no firm evidence on the time frame.

## Answer 149

Sometimes temporary relief is obtained but it depends on the cause of the radiculomyelitis.

## Answer 150

Yes, treat with albendazole although there is little evidence of benefit.
   Patients and the members of their households should be examined for tapeworms. If found, they should be treated with praziquantel 10–20 mg/kg single dose after a light breakfast.

*Further reading*
*(K&C 6e, p. 116.)*
Maguire JH (2004) Tapeworms and seizures – treatment and prevention. *New England Journal of Medicine* **350**: 215–217.

## Answer 151

No, there is no rationale for the use of the drugs mentioned in cerebellar ataxia.

## Answer 152

MRI is characteristic with abnormalities in the subcortical white matter. Genetic analysis (a *NOTCH3* mutation) or a skin biopsy showing granular osmiophilic material (GOM) within small vessels establish the diagnosis. Lactic acid levels are normal.

## Answer 153

This is an interesting point that many have dwelt on over the years. There is no complete understanding of the mechanism.

## Answer 154

Yes, although usually a headache is present.

## Answer 155

The World Health Organization classifies glioblastoma multiforme as grade 4 astrocytomas with endothelial proliferation and necrosis. They also have high mitotic activity. New genetic abnormalities have been described with this tumour.

## Answer 156

Neither acetazolamide nor digoxin are effective.

## Answer 157

The exact existence of normal pressure hydrocephalus, as a true separate entity from dementia, has been questioned. The classic clinical triad is as you have described. MR shows ventriculomegaly but this is also seen in dementia.

## Answer 158

No, you also need to measure the cerebrospinal fluid (CSF) pressure. It is high and CSF can be removed to reduce the pressure.

## Answer 159

Normal CSF pressure is 60–150 mm $H_2O$. CSF pressure is only of diagnostic value in benign intracranial hypertension, in which the figure is greater than 250 mmHg.

## Answer 160

Young children can present with irritability or behavioural disorders rather than headache. Some patients are picked up with papilloedema on examination with no headache.

## Answer 161

No. Sixth nerve palsies can occur.

## Answer 162

Papilloedema is not always present. The frequency will depend on the cause, e.g. papilloedema is rare in raised intracranial pressure associated with hepatic encephalopathy.

## Answer 163

Hyperventilation via intermittent positive-pressure ventilation reduces intracranial pressure by cerebral vasoconstriction within minutes. This is the quickest way to reduce intracranial pressure and is used particularly in unconscious patients who need to be ventilated for respiratory problems.

Mannitol intravenously 1–2 g/kg as a 20% solution over 10–20 minutes reduces cerebral oedema by renal excretion of water. The peak effect is at 90 minutes. It is useful in hepatic failure.

Dexamethasone 10 mg intravenously reduces oedema around a brain tumour or an abscess.

## Answer 164

There is no definite recommendation on the use of anticoagulants. The consensus would probably be not life long.

### Further reading

Stam J (2005) Thrombosis of the cerebral veins and sinuses. *New England Journal of Medicine* **352**: 1791–1798.

## Answer 165
Digoxin has been used but there is little data for its use. Acetazolamide 250 mg × 4 daily, increasing to 500 mg and then 1 g × 4 daily (if tolerated) is the preferred choice.

## Answer 166
Yes, with careful monitoring.

## Answer 167
The relief of symptoms, particularly headache and resolution of visual loss.

## Answer 168
Sudden, acute headache usually associated with intracerebral haemorrhage.

## Answer 169
1. There is no effective treatment/prophylaxis for tension headache, apart from analgesics.
2. Propranolol is of no value.

## Answer 170
All these drugs are antidepressants. They are used in conditions such as tension headaches, particularly if depression is present. Amitriptyline is most often used, but maprotiline and imipramine are as good.

## Answer 171
In 60–70% of cases.

## Answer 172
No. In severe or inadequately controlled hypertension, ergotamine is contraindicated.

## Answer 173
Ergot derivatives are not used often for migraine and they are contraindicated in pregnancy. Use paracetamol.

## Answer 174
Two or more attacks a month that are disabling. Treatment will be for at least a year and long term if necessary.

## Answer 175
Both are used; there are no good comparative studies.

## Answer 176
There are no comparative data and selective serotonin re-uptake inhibitors (SSRIs) have been little used so far in migraine.

## Answer 177

1. Both are used. They have very similar effects.
2. Carbamazepine is not used.

## Answer 178

Verapamil is the only calcium-channel blocker used widely in cluster headaches. In a controlled trial it was as effective as lithium with fewer side-effects.

## Answer 179

Yes, it is worth trying prophylaxis in general practice. Drugs shown to be useful are verapamil, topiramate or lithium. Use whichever drug you are familiar with.

## Answer 180

Ergotamine can be used for patients with short bouts of cluster headaches. However, sumatriptan by SC injection is the drug of choice for treatment.

## Answer 181

There is urinary retention.

## Answer 182

No. A dissociated sensory loss is characteristic with loss of temperature and pain sensation (spinothalamic) with sparing of proprioception and light touch (posterior column).

## Answer 183

It will be initially flaccid at the time of spinal 'shock', then spastic as 'shock' wears off.

## Answer 184

Fasciculations occur with any lower motor neurone lesion, e.g. if a nerve is cut, the muscle it supplies will atrophy and fasciculations occur. Generalized fasciculations are characteristic of motor neurone disease.

## Answer 185

No; there is no convincing evidence of any effect.

## Answer 186

Frontotemporal dementia used to be known as Pick's disease (see K&C 6e, p. 1255). It is often difficult to differentiate it from Alzheimer's disease but characteristically there is much more personality change, disinhibition, and obsessive and compulsive behaviour.

## Answer 187
They do have congenital dislocation of the hips and clubbed feet.

## Answer 188
Yes. Although most are type 2, central neurofibromas can occur in type 1.

## Answer 189
No; unfortunately, there is no effective treatment.

## Answer 190
It has no effect on the heart. NF1 has been associated with a cardiomyopathy.

## Answer 191
a. In lepromatous leprosy the nerves are diffusely and progressively involved, so mononeuritis multiplex is common.
b. 30% of diabetics have a neuropathy, the most common being a motor–sensory neuropathy.

## Answer 192
A positive response produces pain and spasm in the back of the thigh (the hamstrings).

## Answer 193
1. Radiculopathy due to systemic disease can produce a positive stretch test.
2. There is no indication for steroid therapy.

## Answer 194
Disc protrusion, degenerative spinal disease, diabetes and metastatic deposits are some common causes.

## Answer 195
a. It makes it unlikely.
b. Straight leg raising producing pain and limitation is often due to a prolapsed disc with involvement of the sciatic nerve. MRI is the best way to make a diagnosis.

## Answer 196
The paralysis is thought to be due to cross-reacting antibodies to $GM_1$ ganglioside, which is present in high concentrations in the myelin sheath of peripheral nerves. The central spinal fluid usually contains only a few mononuclear cells but has a high protein concentration, sometimes $>5\,g/L$, reflecting immunological rather than infective damage.

## Answer 197
Only *local* steroid injections are used.

## Answer 198
There is no evidence on the value of acetazolamide in the carpal tunnel syndrome.

## Answer 199
As in all scans, the radiologist must know what he or she is looking for.

## Answer 200
Acroparaesthesia does not occur with cervical spondylosis. Beware of false correlations; spondylosis on X-ray is common. The thoracic outlet syndrome produces both vascular and neurogenic symptoms.

## Answer 201
No.

## Answer 202
1. No, this is not a reliable indication. Remember the cord ends at L1, so a paraplegia by definition must occur with a lesion above this and below the cervical region lest a quadriplegia occur.
2. The mechanism is unclear.

## Answer 203
There is no scientific definition of these two terms. 'Asthenia' is an old Greek word describing a lack of strength. 'Weakness' can imply lack of muscle power but is often used to imply tiredness.

## Answer 204
It is not known why many muscle diseases involve proximal rather than distal muscles, causing weakness. In radiculopathies and anterior horn cell disease, the muscles involved depend on which cord level is affected. For example, a disc lesion pressing on L5–S1 produces a distal lesion, whereas involvement of anterior horn cells with polio will affect the muscles of the thigh.

## Answer 205
On electromyography (EMG), spontaneous rhythmic discharges of single muscle fibres are called fibrillations and are not seen clinically. A fasciculation represents a spontaneous discharge of a motor unit, which is seen as a large action potential on EMG and clinically as a muscle twitch. Persistent fasciculation with weakness is seen in motor neurone disease. Myokymia describes a rare continuous, fine, sinous or wave like movement of the lower face that is seen in brainstem lesions, e.g. multiple sclerosis.

## Answer 206

Electromyographic studies show continuous motor activity in the paraspinal muscles in the stiff person syndrome and not in Isaac's syndrome.

## Answer 207

The most common cause is trauma.

## Answer 208

In steroid myopathy the serum creatine phosphokinase (CPK) is normal as is electromyography. Biopsy (usually not necessary) shows type 2 muscle fibre atrophy in steroid-induced myopathy. The CPK is greatly raised in myositis.

## Answer 209

Myositis is a non-suppurative skeletal muscle inflammation. It is often due to a viral cause, e.g. Coxsackie *(see K&C 6e, p. 1267)*.

## Answer 210

Yes it can, and can be confused with myasthenia, which commonly affects these muscles.

## Answer 211

Patients with both chloride channelopathies (e.g. myotonia congenita) and sodium channelopathies (e.g. hyperkalaemic or hypokalaemic periodic paralysis) have been treated with mexilitene. You should not give the drug to patients with bradycardia or high-degree atrioventricular (AV) block (unless the patient has a pacemaker). The major cardiovascular effects are hypotension and arrhythmias, so that electrocardiograms and careful blood pressure monitoring are required. Nausea and vomiting often prevent the drugs being given by mouth.

## Answer 212

No; however, the muscles can be affected to a variable degree so that it can appear to be unilateral.

## Answer 213

The CPK is raised in both myositis and muscle dystrophies. Clinical patterns and electromyography are often more helpful.

## Answer 214

Percussion myotonia – a persistent dimpling after a sharp blow on a muscle, e.g. the thenar eminence or the tongue – is not seen in motor neurone disease. It is seen in myotonia congenita.

## Answer 215
You can't make the diagnosis without papilloedema. CSF pressure measurement is usually performed but repeat lumbar puncture with removal of fluid is used as a treatment.

## Answer 216
Yes; this combination is contraindicated because:
- beta-blockers and thiazide diuretics impair glucose metabolism
- angiotensin-converting enzyme (ACE) inhibitors or antagonists are renoprotective and are therefore first-line treatment in any diabetic.

## Answer 217
Tolosa–Hunt syndrome causes unilateral eye pain, irritation or damage to the IIIrd, IVth or VIth nerves. The pain is relieved by steroids. It is due to cavernous sinus inflammation. CT or MRI will usually show up inflammation.

## Answer 218
1. How long ACTH should be given is unclear; some series suggest months whereas in one big series 75% responded to 2 weeks' therapy.
2. In one study re-administration of ACTH was successful in four out of five patients.

## Answer 219
Steroids are used only for acute attacks of MS. Most studies are with methylprednisolone but dexamethasone has been used with success. 200 mg is a very high dose: 20 mg is more appropriate.

## Answer 220
Yes; aciclovir and steroids should be given together. Trials have shown a benefit.

## Answer 221
You must use corticosteroids for temporal arteritis to prevent blindness. Start prednisolone immediately.

## Answer 222
LDL cholesterol: < 100 mg/dL (2.6 mmol/L). Total: < 4 mmol/L (150 mg/dL).

## Answer 223
Intravenous nitroprusside is rarely necessary even when hypertension is severe. Even with a brain haemorrhage, reduction over 24 hours with oral therapy does less harm than rapid reduction with nitroprusside.

**Answer 224**
Aspirin is contraindicated in someone who has had a previous primary intracerebral haemorrhage.

**Answer 225**
Heubner's artery is a medial lenticulostriate artery that arises from the proximal segment of the anterior communicating artery. It supplies the anterior medial part of the head of the caudate nucleus and the anterior inferior internal capsule. It is identified by surgeons when operating for intracranial aneurysms. There is a spectrum of clinical features of infarction in this area, which partly depends on whether the left or the right side is involved and there are descriptions of predominant weakness of the upper limbs with sparing of the lower limbs in patients with infarction in the territory of Heubner's artery.

**Answer 226**
The view is that statins have a role in plaque stabilization and therefore they are usually given early as you indicate, in the management of myocardial infarction. There is no data on acute management of ischaemic stroke but statins are being used more and more frequently.

**Answer 227**
Captocormia is sometimes called the 'Bent spine syndrome'. It was originally described in a group of servicemen, in whom it was thought to be a psychological reaction to pain. However, this severe forward flexion of the upper spine can occur in several neuro–muscular diseases, e.g. motor neurone disease.

# 22 Psychological medicine

## QUESTIONS

### Question 1
What investigations are recommended in a 70-year-old patient presenting with auditory and visual hallucinations with amnesia?

### Question 2
Could you explain the definitions of pseudohallucinations and quasipsychotic episodes?

### Question 3
What is the 'condensation' and 'displacement' that might underlie formal thought disorder?

### Question 4
Is sulpiride of value in the treatment of conversion disorder?

### Question 5
How does typhoid psychosis manifest? How often does psychosis accompany typhoid fever?

### Question 6
What is the treatment for a case of typhoid psychosis?

### Question 7
Can you please explain to me what changes take place in the body to cause a person to have chronic fatigue syndrome (CFS). I am having difficulty understanding the pathology of this condition.

### Question 8
What is the best treatment for primary insomnia? Could benzodiazepines be used continuously?

## Question 9

Does tolerance develop to the hypnotic effect of trazodone and mianserin? Do these play a role in the treatment of primary insomnia?

## Question 10

Is there a specific treatment for night terror disorders?

## Question 11

Can you suggest possible causes for a 55-year-old female waking regularly at midnight three to four times a month, feeling that she is going to die and feeling an urge to meet people at that time. She has no breathlessness.

## Question 12

What is the modern treatment and prognosis for manic depressive disorder? Is there a malfunction of a metabolic pathway that causes it? Can it be remedied by treatment with neurotransmitter-stimulating drugs? If so which drugs are the most effective apart from lithium carbonate and carbamazepine?

## Question 13

Is lamotrigine as effective a mood stabilizer as lithium?

## Question 14

Is it safe to prescribe lithium for a patient with bipolar mood disorder with biliary cirrhosis and 40% blockage of the main coronary system?

## Question 15

How long should the period of active and maintenance treatment last with mood stabilizers in a patient presenting with his first manic episode?

## Question 16

Do lithium and selective serotonin re-uptake inhibitors (SSRIs) have an anti-impulse effect?

## Question 17

Can any of the antipsychotics clozapine, olanzepine and quetiapine be used as mood stabilizers in bipolar affective disorder?

## Question 18

Is hypothyroidism secondary to chronic lithium therapy in the treatment of bipolar affective disorder, reversible on discontinuation of lithium or its substitution by another mood stabilizer?

## Question 19

In bipolar affective disorder in patients who are well controlled on lithium, is it possible to prescribe thiazide diuretics when hypertension is difficult to control?

## Question 20

Are antipsychotics recommended as the most effective treatment for trichotillomania?

## Question 21

I would like to know when and where antidepressants are used, because I am confused with selective serotonin re-uptake inhibitors (SSRIs), monoamine oxidase inhibitors (MAOIs) and tricyclics.

## Question 22

You have written that the serotonin syndrome results from sudden discontinuation of selective serotonin re-uptake inhibitors (SSRIs) with a short half-life, whereas other books I have read say that serotonin syndrome results from an overdose of SSRI or from combination with monoamine oxidase inhibitors (MAOIs) or serotonin agonists. Please clarify.

## Question 23

What is the safest antipsychotic and antidepressant to give during pregnancy?

## Question 24

How frequently should patients receiving chronic lithium therapy be evaluated for thyroid and renal function?

## Question 25

Is lithium generally associated with bone demineralization, especially in children?

## Question 26

Is lithium recommended in childhood bipolar affective disorder?

## Question 27

Is buspirone as effective as serotonin re-uptake inhibitors (SSRIs) in the treatment of a generalised anxiety disorder?

## Question 28

Can diethylpropion be used to treat children with attention deficit hyperactivity disorder (ADHD)? If so, what is the recommended dose and at what age can it safely be administered?

## Question 29
Can khat (norpseudoephedrine) be given to children with attention deficit hyperactivity disorder and, if so, from what age?

## Question 30
Are selective serotonin re-uptake inhibitors (SSRIs) and venlafaxin effective in the treatment of attention deficit hyperactivity disorder (ADHD)? How efficient are they in comparison with imipramine?

## Question 31
1. Why is weight monitored in infants on methylphenidate for the treatment of attention deficit hyperactivity disorder (ADHD)? Is this to prevent them losing weight, or is losing a certain amount of weight acceptable?
2. Should the electroencephalogram (EEG) be monitored in patients on methylphenidate for ADHD treatment? Should this be stopped if there is some epileptic discharge?

## Question 32
What is the safest typical and atypical antipsychotic, antidepressant and serotonin re-uptake inhibitor (SSRI) used to treat obsessive-compulsive disorder (OCD) that can be used during pregnancy?

## Question 33
What is the rationale for combining serotonin re-uptake inhibitor (SSRIs) and clomipramine in patients with obsessive-compulsive disorder (OCD)? Is this combination more effective than any agent when given alone?

## Question 34
Is sertraline superior to fluoxetine in the treatment of obsessive-compulsive disorder and, if so, why?

## Question 35
I want to find out if there is really a correlation between all cases of delirium tremens (DT) and thiamine deficiency. DT is meant to be a withdrawal state and I assume it can happen in well-nourished alcoholics, as not all alcoholics are malnourished. My friends and I have seen the question that DT is associated with thiamine deficiency in question papers and it has really proved a thorny issue.

## Question 36
1. How long should a doctor treat a patient with the first episode of schizophrenia with regard to the active phase and maintenance therapy?

2. In a patient presenting with the third psychotic episode fulfilling the criteria of schizophrenia, for how long should antipsychotic treatment be continued?

## Question 37

Is there a rationale for treating a patient presenting with his first psychotic episode fulfilling the criteria for schizophrenia, with atypical antipsychotics?

## Question 38

What is the rationale for giving a patient with resistant schizophrenia a combination of typical and atypical antipsychotics?

## Question 39

Do selective serotonin re-uptake inhibitors (SSRIs) have an anti-aggression effect and what is the best anti-aggression drug to be given to schizophrenics and to those suffering from other mental illnesses?

## Question 40

Is depot fluphenazine alone sufficient to treat the active phase of schizophrenia and, if so, what dose is recommended?

## Question 41

Is sulpiride as effective as haloperidol in reducing the positive symptoms of schizophrenia? If yes, what is the most effective dose?

## Question 42

What is the effective daily dose of pimozide? Should it be combined with an anticholinergic? If yes, how long should this combination be continued before giving pimozide on its own?

## Question 43

What percentage of patients receiving chronic conventional antipsychotic treatment develops acute extrapyramidal side-effects and tardive dyskinesia?

## Question 44

How often is risperidone associated with acute extrapyramidal side-effects?

## Question 45

What is the cause of frequent 'freezing' in a schizophrenic patient who shows constant tics and suffers delusions of grandeur, but shows no symptoms of dementia?

## Question 46
Is risperidone more likely to cause tardive dyskinesia than other atypical antipsychotics?

## Question 47
How frequently should patients on clozapine be evaluated for agranulocytosis?

## Question 48
What is meant by 'bipolar spectrum' disorders? Do these include atypical depression and recurrent depressive episodes?

# ANSWERS

## Answer 1
All such patients with new symptoms should have simple blood tests and CT/MRI imaging (Box 22.1).

## Answer 2
Pseudohallucinations are usually auditory and are either true externally sited hallucinations but with insight into their imaginary nature, or are sited within internal space. They do not indicate a psychosis; quasipsychotic is used to describe a type of personality disorder in someone who is not psychotic.

## Answer 3
Condensation is a single symptom or word that is associated with the emotional content of several words.

---

**Box 22.1 Investigations required in a patient suffering from hallucinations with amnesia**

**Blood tests**
- Full blood count
- Erythrocyte sedimentation rate
- Urea and electrolytes
- C-reactive protein
- Blood glucose
- Liver biochemistry
- Serum calcium
- Vitamin $B_{12}$, folate
- Thyroid hormones: thyroid-stimulating hormone, tri-iodothyronine ($T_3$), thyroxine ($T_4$)
- Syphilis serology
- HIV antibodies

**Imaging**
- Chest X-ray
- Computed tomography scan
- Magnetic resonance imaging

**Other**
- Electroencephalogram
- Cerebrospinal fluid
- Brain biopsy

Displacement is a psychological defence mechanism in which there is an unconscious shift of emotions, affect or desires from the original subject to a more acceptable substitute.

## Answer 4
No.

## Answer 5
A psychosis can occur in the third week of a typhoid illness along with apathy and confusion. Typhoid psychosis is unusual. It is described in Ali et al (1997).

*Reference*
Ali G et al. (1997) Spectrum of neuropsychiatric complications in 791 cases of typhoid fever. *Tropical Medicine and International Health* **2**: 314.

## Answer 6
Typhoid psychosis is treated by nursing the patient in a single room. Rehydration is required and the fever is treated with cooling fans and cold water sponging. Appropriate antibiotics are given. Psychoactive drugs should be avoided if possible but in severe psychosis haloperidol 15 mg is the best choice.

## Answer 7
There are no definite pathological features in patients with chronic fatigue syndrome (as most patients don't die of this disease).

## Answer 8
Insomnia is best treated without drugs (*see K&C 6e, p. 1288*). Benzodiazepines, as well as other hypnotics, should only be used for 2 weeks to help relieve an acute situation.

## Answer 9
Mianserin is not a hypnotic and is not used for insomnia. Trazodone is used for insomnia and tolerance does develop.

## Answer 10
Psychotherapy and low-dose benzodiazepines.

## Answer 11
No explanation, I'm afraid!

## Answer 12
Manic depressive disorder is a bipolar disorder in which patients suffer from bouts of depression and mania. The treatment usually involves drugs and the ones you mention are first-line therapy. There is no

definite metabolic pathway malfunction in manic depressive disorder.

## Answer 13
No, lamotrigine is not as effective as lithium.

## Answer 14
With careful monitoring, lithium could, if indicated, be used in such a patient.

## Answer 15
Six months after the first episode in bipolar disorders. There is a case, however, to continue for 2 years as relapse is high. Withdrawal of lithium should be slow because of evidence of rebound mania.

## Answer 16
DSM-IV-TR describes an impulse disorder as 'the failure to resist an impulse, drive or temptation to commit an act that is harmful to the individual and others'. Both lithium and SSRIs have been effective in individual patients. There are no trials.

## Answer 17
Antipsychotics have been used as second- or third-line therapy particularly in acute mania. They should only be used by experts in the field.

## Answer 18
It is usually reversible.

## Answer 19
Both loop and thiazide diuretics reduce the excretion of lithium, and increase the plasma concentrations of lithium with consequent toxicity occur. This is more severe with thiazide diuretics, which should be avoided. This is a difficult problem, which might require a change of therapy.

## Answer 20
The most effective treatment is cognitive behavioural therapy and a selective serotonin re-uptake inhibitor; this is the treatment of first choice.

## Answer 21
Tricyclic antidepressants are still commonly used as first-line pharmacotherapy in patients with depression. They have been available for many years and are therefore familiar to many practitioners. Tricyclic-related drugs, e.g. trazodone, have a lower incidence of antimuscarinic effects (e.g. constipation and dry mouth), common side-effects of tricyclics.

The SSRIs, e.g. paroxetine, also have fewer antimuscarinic effects and are safe in overdose, although no more effective than tricyclics. They are being used more and more in the same situations for which you would use tricyclics.

MAOIs, e.g. phenelzine have interactions with other drugs and some foods and are much less commonly used, except by experienced physicians usually when tricyclics are ineffective.

## Answer 22

'Serotonin syndrome' is a toxic hyperserotonergic state. It is, as you say, typically the result of combining a serotonergic agent with a monoamine oxidase inhibitor (*see K&C 6e, p. 1292*). This is, however, not always the case (see Sternbach 1991). Remember: there is also a 'discontinuity syndrome' and patients must reduce SSRIs slowly.

*Reference*
Sternbach H (1991) The serotonin syndrome. *American Journal of Psychiatry* **148**: 705–713.

## Answer 23

Conventional 'typical' antipsychotics, e.g. promazine, haloperidol. Selective serotonin re-uptake inhibitors, e.g. paroxetine, are the safest for depression in pregnancy. All drugs must only be given if absolutely necessary in pregnancy.

## Answer 24

Every 3–6 months.

## Answer 25

No.

## Answer 26

Yes. Several short-term studies show benefit.

## Answer 27

SSRIs or venlafaxine are first line-treatments. Buspirone is the second choice.

## Answer 28

No. Diethylpropion should not be used under 12 years of age and there are no data on its use in ADHD.

## Answer 29

It might help but the only accepted drugs used in this condition are methylphenidate and atomoxetine. They should not be used under 6 years of age.

## Answer 30
Desipramine 200 mg daily has been shown to be better than a placebo. SSRIs are not helpful, but studies are small.

## Answer 31
1. Anorexia and weight loss occur and weight should be monitored.
2. EEG monitoring is not normally required but methylphenidate should not be given to epileptics.

## Answer 32
OCD should be treated with cognitive behavioural therapy (CBT), and drugs should be avoided in pregnancy. If drug treatment is essential, an SSRI, e.g. paroxetine, should be used.

## Answer 33
SSRIs have replaced clomipramine; there is no rationale for combining the two.

## Answer 34
Both are SSRIs and are probably of similar effect.

## Answer 35
Thiamin deficiency is not a cause of DT, which is part of the withdrawal state, and many patients who suffer from it are severe alcoholics who may well be thiamin deficient. It is therefore advised that thiamine be given to the patient but not directly for the management of DT.

## Answer 36
1. Long-term treatment of a patient who definitely has schizophrenia is frequently necessary even after one episode. This is because withdrawal of treatment can produce severe relapses, which occur at unpredictable intervals. Therefore, long-term maintenance therapy is required.
2. Certainly, after three psychotic episodes, lifetime therapy would be indicated; withdrawal would only be done under very careful supervision.

## Answer 37
There is more and more emphasis on using the so-called atypical antipsychotics. Risperidone at a starting dose of 2 mg twice daily increasing to 10 mg daily would be a commonly used drug.

## Answer 38
The only time this should happen is when an atypical antipsychotic is being added to eventually replace the typical drug. By and large, there is no advantage in giving more than one drug in schizophrenia.

## Answer 39
SSRIs are not useful as an anti-aggressive drug. The best treatment is zuclopenthixol acetate 50–150 mg by deep IM injection.

## Answer 40
Fluphenazine, initially 2.5–10 mg rising to 20 mg daily, can be used but extrapyramidal symptoms are a problem. There is a move to use so-called 'atypical antipsychotics' instead.

## Answer 41
Yes, possibly better. A high dose of sulpiride is needed: 2.4 g daily.

## Answer 42
Start with 2 mg daily, increasing at weekly intervals up to 16 mg if necessary.
   Routine antimuscarinics are not justified because not all patients have side-effects, and they may unmask or worsen tardive dyskinesia.

## Answer 43
Over 50% will get side-effects, usually reversible.

## Answer 44
We can't give a figure but less often than with the usual antipsychotic drugs.

## Answer 45
'Freezing' occurs in schizophrenia but the mechanism is unclear. However, positron emission tomography (PET) scan studies show abnormalities in dopamine receptors.

## Answer 46
No; at low daily doses (<6 mg) extrapyramidal side-effects are uncommon.

## Answer 47
White cell count every week for 18 weeks; every 2 weeks up to 1 year; then monthly.

## Answer 48
Bipolar disorders are divided into two subgroups:
- a history of one manic episode with or without a depressive episode
- a history of at least one depressive episode and one hypomanic episode.

The term embraces the whole spectrum of mania with or without depression but is not used for depression alone.

# 23 Skin disease

**Question 1**
Other than *Staphylococcus aureus*, which pathogens cause furuncles?

**Question 2**
Can a skin disease, in particular a fungal disease, cause enlarged, tender lymph nodes?

**Question 3**
In a 5-month-old baby with eczema:
1. What is the best treatment?
2. What is the prognosis?
3. What is the benefit of cleaning the affected areas with cold water?

**Question 4**
Does psoriasis cause the formation of hypopigmented patches?

**Question 5**
What is the suggested treatment for black spots on the face? What is the latest recommended treatment for acne?

**Question 6**
1. Are there any side-effects from long-term use (2–3 months) of a topical antibiotic for acne vulgaris?
2. Is folliculitis related to the condition or the treatment in any way?

**Question 7**
Is there a diagnostic test for acne rosacea? If intermittent facial flushing occurs on a regular basis, what other diagnosis might be reached?

## Question 8
Where can I find a model algorithm for the investigation of pruritus?

## Question 9
I would like to ask why moles form, particularly on the skin of the face. What is their non-surgical treatment?

## Question 10
In a patient with malignant melanoma, what do the following increasing values of thymidine kinase (mitotic index = 2; Breslow = 3; Clark = 4) predict?

## Question 11
What prognosis can be expected when a malignant melanoma is diagnosed with the results of Clark 4 and Breslow 3?

## Question 12
I have been wondering about the colouring of the skin in patients with haemochromatosis. You write 'bronze skin pigmentation (due to melanin deposition)', but I can't understand where the increased melanin comes from? An increased production of melanin-stimulating hormone (MSH) doesn't seem to fit in well with the decreased function of the gland regarding other hormones.

## Question 13
Please explain how to make a positive identification of vitiligo. I would be grateful if you could suggest further reading material for this condition.

## Question 14
Can a shagreen patch in tuberous sclerosis be bluish in colour?

## Question 15
What medical and minimally invasive therapy is available in Pakistan and in India for palmar hyperhidrosis?

## Question 16
Some people suffer with a non-hairy beard, others with fine and scanty hair. What treatment would you advise for both extremes?

## Question 17
Can alopecia universalis be due to psychological problems?

## ANSWERS

### Answer 1
*Staphylococcus aureus* is the only common cause of furuncles.

### Answer 2
No.

### Answer 3
1. Emollients to hydrate the skin. Topical steroids (low potency) are also helpful.
2. Good. It usually clears.
3. Better to use emollients *(see K&C 6e, p. 1364)*.

### Answer 4
Yes; particularly with topical treatment.

### Answer 5
There are many causes of black spots, including the blackheads seen in acne. Treatment for mild to moderate acne is still topical, e.g. benzoyl peroxide, antibiotics, retinoids; with oral antibiotics for moderate/severe disease, e.g. minocycline 100 mg daily, or hormone treatment, e.g. co-cyprindiol in females. Very severe disease is treated with oral retinoids. These are teratogenic and their use is restricted to being supervised by a dermatologist.

### Answer 6
1. Local irritation occurs but generally topical antibiotics are safe. *Propionibacterium acnes*-resistant strains occur.
2. Folliculitis is a pyoderma localized to hair follicles and is not related to acne.

### Answer 7
No; it is a clinical diagnosis. The flushing may precede the other signs by a number of years.

### Answer 8
This model is given in Fig. 23.1, which is derived from Table 23.9 on p. 1345 of Kumar and Clark *Clinical Medicine* 6th edn.

### Answer 9
Moles can appear anywhere on the body, but just seem to be more prevalent on the face. There is no other treatment than removal. Cosmetic therapy can be tried.

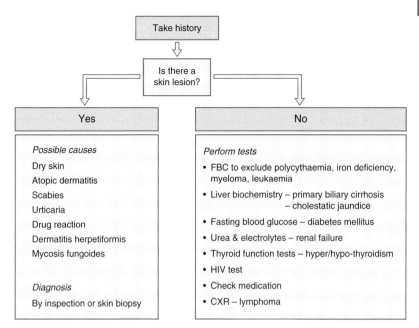

**Fig. 23.1** Model algorithm for the investigation of pruritus. CXE, chest X-ray; FBC, full blood count; HIV, human immunodeficiency virus.

## Answer 10
Thymidine kinase is increased during DNA synthesis in cell proliferation. Increasing thickness is associated with increased recurrence: those with tumour less than 1 mm thick have an 80–90% 10-year survival. Increasing level of invasion (Clark's level) and a high mitotic rate are poor prognostic factors.

## Answer 11
Between 40 and 50% 10-year survival is a general figure. You need careful staging with TNM to accurately predict prognosis.

*Further reading*
Thompson JF et al (2007) Case 2–2007 Malignant melanoma. *New England Journal of Medicine* **356:** 285–292.

## Answer 12
Bronze skin pigmentation is due to both iron and melanin deposition. It is not related to increased production of adrenocorticotrophic hormone or MSH.

## Answer 13
Vitiligo is an acquired destruction of melanocytes giving white patches on the skin. The lesions are usually well defined and sometimes have a hyperpigmented margin.

*Further reading*
Grimes PE (2005) New insights and new therapies on vitiligo. *Journal of the American Medical Association* **293:** 730–735.

## Answer 14
They are normally flesh coloured.

## Answer 15
Alpha-adrenergic-blocking drugs such as phenoxybenzamine have been used, as has propantheline, with varying success. Injection of Botox directly into the palms reduces sweating but it is painful and expensive. Sympathetic denervation by resection of the 2nd thoracic sympathetic ganglion can be performed with minimal invasive surgery. Sweating is stopped initially but it returns.

## Answer 16
In both cases, treatment is cosmetic.

## Answer 17
The cause is unknown. Psychological problems have been implicated.

# Index